MW01601910

VEGAN KETO & INTERMITTENT FASTING

THE EASY 4-STEP / 4-WEEK METHOD TO LOSE
WEIGHT, DETOX YOUR BODY AND BOOST
YOUR ENERGY. INCLUDES: 4-WEEK VEGAN
MEAL PLAN AND 37 TASTY KETO RECIPES.

TAKALANI BRIDGET N.

Written by
MEGAN MCCOIG

Sourc

CONTENTS

INTRODUCTION

Welcome to the ultimate guide for Vegan Keto & Intermittent Fasting diet! The easy step by step method for those who want to start a keto diet while remaining 100% vegan.

This book will be your guide to help you begin your new lifestyle change. We will cover all bases and information needed about diet requirements, benefits, and more.

With there being an abundance of new diets worldwide, it may be overwhelming for some. So, we have covered all the relevant research and information you will need to successfully fulfill a true vegan keto diet.

Throughout the book, each diet technique and information will be discussed. This will help you understand the science, restrictions, and rules behind each diet. It will also give you an understanding of exactly how each diet can benefit the body. Then collectively, this book will guide you into putting the diets altogether to optimize your health, and eating desires.

We will begin with Intermittent Fasting. A method that integrates fasting into the diet for amazing health benefits.

Then, we will discuss veganism. Lovers of the environment and sustainable living are usually vegan. Eliminating the slaughtering and consumption of animal products is helping the world.

To look after our bodies, we should manage our weight and balance our lifestyle habits. Caring for both your mind and for your body is as important as one another.

For those who want to care for the world as much as their body, veganism is the answer. A more sustainable and healthier way to eat is a plant-based diet. Choosing plant-based alternatives is one step closer to saving the world. and being part of veganism.

Second, we will inform you about the keto diet. Many pursue this diet to limit carb intake for multiple health reasons.

Although it can be difficult to sustain a healthy diet without overconsuming carbohydrates whilst being vegan, it is achievable. A simple answer to reducing carbohydrate intake is to limit your daily intake. How to do that, whilst maintaining a balanced diet, is what this book is for. The carbohydrate-restricted diet is better known as the Keto Diet.

The benefits of the keto diet are phenomenal due to the limitation of carbohydrates. This diet is heavy in animal products in most cases. But, this book will help you understand it is easy to consume a Keto Diet whilst being 100% vegan.

Most people assume that health conditions such as obesity, heart disease, and diabetes are a result of high-fat foods. But, the main culprit is sugar. Sugar is in almost everything humans eat, especially foods high in carbohydrates.

High carbohydrate foods include dairy, grains, legumes,

starchy vegetables, and sugary treats. All of which are equally as high in sugar. These foods are in fact, all to be either eliminated or reduced on the keto diet whilst being vegan.

The risk of heart conditions is better reduced by limiting your carbohydrate intake. More so than the consumption of animal products, due to the high sugar content. Both do contribute to heightening the risk of many diseases and detrimental illnesses.

Your body can be healthier by partaking in a keto vegan diet. The combination of both diets also encourages the world to be more sustainable. Veganism is a way of life to be proud of and you should not limit yourself to eating only carbs. The vegan keto diet offers an extensive list of delicious foods. This includes high-fat foods, plant-based proteins, and low carbohydrate options. All, packed full of flavor and nutrition.

Do not worry about getting all the essential nutrients whilst being on the diet, we will cover it all. From foods to supplements, encouragement, and recipes, this book has it all.

This book will be your holy grail if you want to know how to fulfill the keto diet whilst being vegan. It will also help you achieve a healthy weight and a healthy mind.

Being on a vegan diet may make other diet techniques seem difficult or unachievable. With the right food substitutes, you can achieve a healthy and successful keto vegan diet. Having set meal plans and routines are helpful too. If you wish to try intermittent fasting whilst being on a Keto vegan diet, that is very beneficial.

If your goal is to lose weight whilst being vegan, the keto diet is a great solution.

You may wonder how to sustain a keto diet whilst being free from animal products such as meat, dairy, and eggs. The keto diet allows for animal products. But, for vegans, there are alternatives for this. This includes substitutes such as plant-based proteins and dairy-free foods.

There is no need to worry about nutritional deficiencies as there are many solutions. This book will cover everything you need to ensure safety. With the right knowledge, it is easy to avoid risks and health concerns. A lack of knowledge may result in poor health, so it is important to understand before starting.

A lack of understanding can pose risks and side effects. Such as muscular issues, severe weakness, and vitamin deficiencies (1).

Use this book as your guide. It will help you understand the keto diet and intermittent fasting. It will help you understand how to make the diet sustainable and risk-free whilst being vegan.

I have been a nutritionist for many years. I have tested the keto and intermittent fasting diets on many clients. Many of whom were vegan or vegetarian. The test results have helped me perfect the best plan for being on the diets whilst being vegan.

Sharing my faultless knowledge will help you win this time. It will help you lose weight and sustain a healthy keto diet whilst being 100% vegan. You can also add in intermittent fasting without being at risk.

You may be wondering more about me. My name is Takalani Bridget Netshiomvani. In 2005 I completed my studies at the University of Venda with a BSc degree in nutrition. Over the years as a nutritionist, I have helped many people reach their weight loss goals. I have tested many diets to find the best ones for weight loss. I have helped all my clients achieve their body goals through menu planning and diets.

For long term results, the combination of two diets is very effective. In particular, the keto diet and intermittent fasting are one of the most beneficial.

If you want some proof of the results, here is more.

My vegan clients who were struggling to lose weight found the keto vegan diet very effective. All reported amazing results and lifestyle changes due to this diet.

Many vegans rely on carbohydrate-heavy foods to sustain energy and see it as an easy alternative. This is a very lazy way to eat. There are plenty of delicious and exciting foods out there for the keto vegan diet.

Those who followed the keto vegan diet and intermittent fasting saw a weight loss of around 9 pounds. The funny fact is that they also convinced their partners to try the diet and the majority enjoyed it too.

People see incredible results from this diet. They all started the diet with no concern and all achieved their goals. It makes you realize that the sooner you start, the sooner you will achieve your goals. The sooner you start, the quicker you will see results.

A client of mine reported back to me, "When I did vegan keto for about 2 months, I shed like 30lbs. It was wild. I also did intermittent fasting which I'm sure helped. But the weight fell off so fast."

Whilst another said, "Still losing, 55lbs down so far since June 14th of this year. High carb low fat is exactly what led to me continuing to gain weight and feeling hungry all the time. Eating at a caloric deficit is easy on the keto vegan diet. I don't have many cravings which are making weight loss easier. Plus, there are all sorts of perks from the Keto Diet such as improved sleep, clearer skin, more energy, etc."

Based on a keto vegan diet with intermittent fasting, there are many health benefits. This includes improving weight loss, heart health, and neurological diseases. It can also help inhibit or slow the progression of cancer and diabetes (2).

So, I've decided to share with you my ultimate guide, meal plan, recipes, health benefits and so much more in this book. All chapters will answer the questions you may have about the keto vegan diet. Everything in here will help you get started on your journey sooner, rather than later.

You may wonder what you will gain from reading this book and trying out the 4-week plan. The first thing you will gain is the results. By following this program, my client base lost an average of 8 to 10 pounds.

The diet is easier when people understand what foods they should and should not eat. Over time, the diet will become a natural part of your daily routine. When you start to notice amazing results, it'll encourage you to stick to it. Why wouldn't you want to stick to a diet that makes you feel and look amazing?

The majority of my clients report it takes around 2-3 weeks of being on the diet for it to feel natural. The foods and meal plans will become a natural part of your routine too. Most people never turn back to a non-keto vegan diet.

Not only will you gain plenty of understanding of the diet, but you will also reap many health benefits. I will be sharing more about the health benefits later on and in more depth. For now, it is important to acknowledge that the diet has many health benefits that can benefit all.

After reading this book and completing 4 weeks of a keto vegan diet, you will gain a new healthier lifestyle. You will also find out your favorite recipes, foods, and will be independent for the rest of your journey. You will be your own master of the diet and what works for you. You will know how to face nutrient deficiencies and the intermittent fasting windows. And of course, you will lose weight and enjoy it.

Here is my promise to you.

With my help, you will gain the skills and knowledge you need to sustain a keto vegan diet and fast at the same time.

Reaching your weight goal and a healthier lifestyle will be easy to achieve with this book. By following the 4-week program you will reach your body and mind goals. The book will expand your knowledge and help you achieve the ideal diet plan. In time, sticking to the plan will help you sustain the diet long term.

Do you ever question a new lifestyle choice and wonder what you would be feeling like now if you'd started it a year ago? Imagine how you would feel now if you started the diet the day you thought about starting it, instead of waiting.

Many of us find it easy to leave a task until tomorrow. That delay in getting it done then prolongs to the next day, then the next and then the next. Putting something off is not going to get you results neither is it a healthy mindset.

There is no need to delay getting started with the new diet. Once you have read the book and attained all the information you need, you can begin.

Reading this book and following the curated 4-week program will make you your own master of the diet.

The keto diet and intermittent fasting is both manageable and sustainable whilst being 100% vegan. Continue reading to find out more about the diet, its benefits, and the 4-week program.

Your first day can be now and today. So let the diet begin to get started, achieve results, and influence sustainability.

BEFORE READING

You will find all sources, updates, links and bonuses on our dedicated page :

fcer.org/vegan-keto-IF-book/

Don't forget to connect to this page with the password (find it on the « Access to the online area » part) to get access to all the free bonuses.

PART I

INTERMITTENT FASTING 101

« Fasting is the first principle of medicine; fast and see the strength of the spirit reveal itself. »

— Rumi

1

WHAT IS INTERMITTENT FASTING?

Many people assume that fasting is starvation. That assumption is incorrect. Starvation is an involuntary uncontrolled period without food. Whereas fasting is voluntary and controlled. Fasting, especially intermittent fasting, is for health, religious and spiritual reasons.

Intermittent fasting is an eating pattern method with cycled mealtimes. The method is often shortened to "IF". It does not dictate which foods to eat and avoid. Instead, it gives you time periods of eating and not eating. The technique provides meal time cycles.

Understanding how to intermittent fast is essential so that a person does not over fast. Lack of knowledge can be damaging to the body and the mind.

The fasting technique is often used to aid weight loss. The food cycles allow your body to use and burn fat quicker. This helps speed up the process of weight loss and improves body fat mass and BMI. Not only does it help with weight management, it offers many more health benefits. Fasting can improve heart health, brain function, and lifespan. It can also slow the progression of medical conditions such as diabetes, cancer, and aging.

Many people who contemplate fasting worry that it can cause health risks. Many worry that the cons may outweigh the pros. Intermittent fasting offers more health benefits than it does risks.

For the majority, fasting is nourishing and safe for the body. It is a detoxifying ritual that the body benefits from, more than it does from eating too much or too often. The human body can withstand periods of fasting and lack of food. Ever since times of war, plagues and epidemics humans have had to practice fasting and periods of no food at all.

Throughout history, fasting was a useful way for humans to ration food. This rationing inhibited supplies from being completely used up. Today, fasting is a healthy and natural way for the body to detoxify and regenerate.

Due to its history, scientists have a newfound understanding of intermittent fasting. They acknowledge that it is sustainable by the human body. Investigations have looked into its health benefits and risks. More of which, we will share later. It is important to be aware that intermittent fasting can pose benefits and risks. Yet, risks are very limited.

The most common concern is the lack of food and essential nutrients. In some cases, nutritional deficiencies can occur. But, people can replace these nutrients with supplements. This is easy to avoid if a person sticks to nutritional and balanced meals.

The intermittent fasting techniques have no set duration. The most popular intermittent fasting method is 16:8. This is where a person does not eat for 16 hours of the day and eats for the remaining 8 hours. This time rationed meal cycle is better known as time-restricted eating. This is because it dictates periods of when you eat. There are alternative cycles which include 14:10 and 12:12. The first number indicates the fasting hours and the second, the eating hours.

There more are intermittent fasting methods. Including alternate day fasting, meal skipping, 5:2, and eat stop eat. This book will share each method and their process which will help you decide which method is best for you.

Many people choose a method based on their current diet and lifestyle. The majority choose the one most suitable and beneficial for their health. Many do not understand quite how intermittent fasting works. So, here is more.

HOW DOES INTERMITTENT FASTING WORK?

T here are 5 stages to intermittent fasting. Each stage allows the body to go through a repairing process. All stages promote slowing the progression of diseases to inhibiting health conditions.

The body adjusts on a cellular and molecular level due to a change in hormones. This includes the ghrelin hormone which works to suppress and control hunger. These hunger hormones work to make stored body fat accessible.

Stage 1. 12 hours - Ketosis

Energy comes from foods that are high in carbohydrates. These foods include grains, legumes, starchy vegetables, and wheat products. All of which are high in glucose, which is where the energy comes from. When there is no longer any glucose to use as fuel due to fasting, the body looks for other sources of fuel. That secondary source is 'stored' fat. Ketosis is the process where the body sources other energy due to lack of glucose.

Ketosis involves the body using fat as fuel. This usually happens after 12 hours of fasting and encourages fat loss. Fat burning increases during fasting. The fat-burning benefit is well known as one of the key benefits of intermittent fasting.

Stage 2. 24 hours - Autophagy

Cells begin to repair when the body adjusts to hunger controlling hormones. The cells repair from previous food intake and exercise. This is better known as autophagy and is the process where old cells digest, diminish, and then renew. Autophagy is a natural way for the body to remove dysfunctional cells. It helps replace the old cells with new healthier cells full of protein.

Autophagy can only begin when glucose and insulin levels are low. It is a healthy process for cells and tissue to repair. It can inhibit medical conditions and neurological diseases. Studies suggest autophagy begins after 24 hours of calorie restrictions. It can increase with exercise during periods of fasting (3).

Stage 3. 48 hours - Growth hormones increase

Throughout fasting, the body's human growth hormones (HGH) increase. Fasting enhances the growth of hormones. In particular, the human growth hormones increase at an exponential rate. The increase of hormone secretion contributes to many health benefits. This includes weight loss, fat burning and muscle gain.

Also to this, the body's ghrelin hormone increases. This hormone controls hunger and suppresses appetite. These two processes are beneficial for weight loss and management. It also helps to build lean muscle and reduce fat tissue.

Stage 4. 54 hours - Insulin balance

After 54 hours, the body learns to balance insulin levels. During fasting, the body sees huge changes in insulin. The fasting period allows the body to digest food better. This helps improve insulin sensitivity and reduces insulin levels.

Studies show how lower insulin levels help stored fat be more accessible (4). This is often called fat burning. Fat burning encourages weight loss. It also improves a person's ability to maintain a healthier weight, fat mass, and BMI. Fat burning is very beneficial for diabetic patients. Especially those who have type 2 diabetes as insulin sensitivity is a huge medical issue (5).

Stage 5. 72 hours - Immune cell rejuvenation

After 72 hours, immune cells begin to rejuvenate. This process enhances gene expression. Many studies have shown how fasting can cause gene expression. Gene expression refers to changes in the genes.

This process reduces the risk of developing health conditions. It can reduce the development of conditions such as cancer and brain aging. Thus, gene expression has benefits for healthier life-long living. This includes life longevity and protecting the body against disease and illness (6).

After the body has gone through all 5 stages, it is time to refeed the body. It is important to break a fast with nutritious balanced foods. Foods low in carbohydrates and sugar are best for easing your body back into digestion.

Balanced foods will improve cell function and replenish the body with what it will need.

These 5 stages are significant for the health benefits offered by intermittent fasting. Whilst the body fasts and goes from a state of ketosis to cell rejuvenation, the body benefits in a variety of ways.

INTERMITTENT FASTING BENEFITS

With intermittent fasting comes many health benefits. People associate diets and intermittent fasting with weight loss. But, there are many other health benefits a person can gain from intermittent fasting. From improved heart health to reduce the chance of inflammation and cancers.

1 - Encourages Weight Loss

The number one benefit of intermittent fasting is weight loss. Yet, intermittent fasting focuses on more than that.

Intermittent fasting is a simple way to reduce calorie intake for most. This is due to the cycle of eating and fasting. The cycle can reduce body weight, improve body composition and increase metabolism.

When the body is fasting, energy comes from stored fat instead of glucose. The human body uses food eaten throughout the day for energy. But, if fasting is in place and no food is being consumed, it has to seek energy elsewhere. The first solution for that is using fat for fuel. Fat burning encourages incredible weight management benefits.

Scientists review intermittent fasting as a great solution to reduce obesity levels. Science suggests many can enjoy fasting to reduce weight and body fat. It can also improve their body composition (7).

2 - Reduces Insulin Resistance

Intermittent fasting is great for reducing insulin resistance. This is beneficial and ideal for diabetic patients. Insulin rises during eating to help store the food and its nutrients as energy. The fasting process reduces the need to store fuel as fat which helps the insulin level balance out.

Studies show a reduction in insulin levels from low-calorie intake via fasting. The fasting window allows the body to use up stored glucose and fat as energy. This inhibits glucose overload, which helps decline insulin levels and resistance. It is good for the body to have time to digest food. It helps to use up stored fat for energy and burn fat quicker.

Intermittent fasting can also reduce blood sugar levels. Studies reveal how it can lower blood sugar levels by up to 6% with calorie control. Then, up to 31% with intermittent fasting (8).

3 - Helps Increase Heart Health

Intermittent fasting is profound for having many benefits for the heart. Studies show how patients who IF have lower LDL cholesterol, which is the bad cholesterol. It can also lower blood sugar levels and reduce triglycerides. Both contribute to good heart health.

For those with poor health, intermittent fasting has

positive effects. Such as obese or diabetic individuals. But, everyone can reap this benefit. For those who are heart-healthy, it can maintain good heart health.

4 - Reduces Inflammation

Many chronic diseases are due to inflammation. This includes asthma, arthritis, bowel issues, and neurological conditions. Intermittent fasting can benefit Alzheimer's disease and dementia patients (9).

Studies for intermittent fasting show incredible results for its anti-inflammatory benefits. Anyone that chooses intermittent fasting can gain anti-inflammatory benefits.

5 - Increases Brain Health

Intermittent fasting has proved to increase the brain-derived neurotrophic factor hormone. This hormone is better known as BDNF. The diet restrictions encourage the growth of the hormone. The lack of food produces BDNF and is then sent to the brain and increases brain health.

BDNF plays a vital role in decreasing the risk of Alzheimer's disease, science suggests. The BDNF hormone helps protect the brain from developing neurological diseases.

Science proves that the BDNF hormone plays a vital role in neuronal growth and survival (10). It is an essential neurotransmitter that enhances memory and learning. The increase of BDNF is essential from a young age to help with good function and growth. Intermittent fasting can boost BDNF in young adults.

6 - May Prevent Cancer

Fasting for large periods has shown to have impressive results for preventing cancers. In particular, fasting plays a role in decreasing tumors that may lead to cancer. It can also slow down the progression of such conditions.

So far the testing has been complete on animals, but in most cases, animal testing does prove to be true for humans too (11).

The testing has not yet signified which cancers it can inhibit or slow down the progression of. Yet, research shows that intermittent fasting can reverse the effects of cancer.

7 - Offers Anti-aging Properties

A test on rats showed that intermittent fasting can extend life span by up to 83%. A positive correlation between growth and longer life span was a result of the testing. This suggests that intermittent fasting will have a similar effect on adults (12).

It seems that again, the dietary restrictions played a key role in these tests. Among the participants, fasting with calorie restrictions resulted in a longer lifespan.

There are several different types of intermittent fasting. Each method offers similar health benefits. But, all abide by different restrictions and rules.

4

5 TYPES OF INTERMITTENT FASTING

There are many intermittent fasting methods a person can try. Yet, not all are safe or effective. All methods have different effects on the body and results.

It can help most people to try a few different methods to understand what will work best for them.

All intermittent fasts include not eating for a certain period of that time. In the window where you do not eat, water and calorie-free drinks such as black tea and coffee are fine to consume.

To save you time and danger, below are the top 5 intermittent fasting methods. These are all proven to be safe, effective, and beneficial for various health reasons.

1 - The Time-Restricted Eating Method - 16:8

The time-restricted eating method is one of the most popular dieting methods used today. It seems to be the most lifestyle-friendly and easiest to follow. This is because it is safe to do every day or other day.

The most popular time-restricted eating intermittent fast is 16:8. This is where a person fasts for 16 hours and eats in the remaining 8 hours. It can be as simple as not eating anything after dinner and skipping breakfast.

During the timed fast, it is common to drink calorie-free drinks as it can help reduce hunger. Yet, no food or calories. It is good for your energy levels to stay hydrated throughout the fast. Thus, choose water over dehydrating options as and when you can.

It is important to not overeat when you break your fast and throughout your eating window. Overconsumption of food will decrease results, especially for those seeking weight loss.

The idea of a smaller window to eat means a person will often eat 2 meals a day and a snack as opposed to 3 meals a day. Those 2 meals may sometimes be bigger in size but should always be nutritious if you wish to reap the benefits. The same goes for if you want the fast to be effective.

The alternate time-restricted eating methods, which in ratio format such as 16:8, include 12:12 and 14:10. The first number dictates the hours you do not eat for then, the latter indicates the window you should use to eat.

You can choose what times to stop and start eating. For example, you can stop eating at 8.p.m and begin again at 12.p.m the next day for the 16 hour fast. This then means you can eat for 8 hours between 12.p.m and 8.p.m. Or, you can stop at 5.p.m and start eating again at 9 am the next day. It is up to the person, their preference and lifestyle. As long as you stick to the fasting window, you will complete the time-restricted eating period.

2 - The Twice A Week Method - 5:2

Another popular method of intermittent fasting is the 5:2 diet. Sometimes referred to as the twice a week fasting method. This involves fasting/calorie restriction for 2 days of the week. The 2 fasting days should expect a person to eat around 500 to 600 calories. This should be two small meals of 250 to 300 calories each as opposed to one meal. Eating two smaller meals will reduce fatigue that may occur.

For the remaining 5 days of the week, a person can consume their recommended calorie amount. They should also stick to nutritious balanced meals to avoid excessive eating. For those seeking weight loss, calories should not be excessive on normal eating days. Excessive eating may result in weight gain.

Scientific research shows how the 5:2 method can be very beneficial for weight loss and gut health. This method is often reported to be sustainable and effective. Even more so when the meals you do consume are healthy and nutritious.

3 - The 24 Hour/Water Method - Eat Stop Eat

The 'eat stop eat' intermittent fasting method may seem the hardest out of them all. It involves 24 hours of complete fasting with only water allowed.

For most people, it is common to fast from dinner one day to dinner time the following day. This means the person would complete an entire 24 hours of fasting. But, the 24 hour fast can be from breakfast to breakfast or lunch to lunch as well.

Many recommend to only do the 'eat stop eat' method only once or twice a week. Those days are dependent on the individual and their preference. This is because this method can cause extreme side effects. It can cause extreme fatigue, very low energy, irritability, and headaches.

Like the other fasts, calorie-free drinks are fine but not solid foods or calories.

It may be best to try other intermittent fasting methods before trying the 'eat stop eat' method. This will help a person avoid extreme side effects and risks. It will also allow them to understand if fasting is sustainable for them.

After fasting, return to the normal eating routine and calorie intake.

4 - The Spontaneous Method: Meal Skipping

Not all intermittent fasting plans involve fasting for long periods. Some methods, like meal skipping, can allow a person to reap some of the amazing health benefits.

The meal skipping method involves spontaneous meal skipping throughout the day.

Many assume that the human body needs feeding every few hours or every single mealtime, that is not true. But, science proves that humans can deal with meal skipping.

This intermittent fasting method involves skipping random meals throughout the week. Meal skipping allows your digestive system to have a break and to break down food better. It helps aid better digestion.

Many may find this method easier, to begin with as it is easier to fast for a smaller amount of time. If you would like to try longer fasting periods it is best to ease yourself into it. Try starting with the meal skipping technique to help your body adjust.

5 - The Every Other Day Method - Alternate Day Fasting

The alternate-day fasting method involves modified fasting every other day.

For some, the fasting day involves 24 hours of fasting. Then, for others, they allow themselves to consume up to 500 calories. The time-restricted eating windows such as 16:8 can work here too.

For example, alternate days will see a person eat their normal meals and calorie intake. The remaining days will focus on a 24 hour fast or calorie restrictions.

Studies show that this method does work but has less effect. Especially for weight control and reducing blood sugar level/ cholesterol than other methods.

Most methods that involve restricting calorie intake results in weight loss. But, it is important to not overcompensate for the loss of calories during the windows of eating. Otherwise, the results may not be as evident.

Many choose the time-restricted eating method of 16:8 as intermittent fasting. This is because it concludes to be the most effective and beneficial for weight loss and more.

5

THE 16:8 METHOD

The 16:8 method is the most popular in intermittent fasting. For this reason, we must cover all areas to help those interested in trying this. It will also benefit those who wish to make it a part of their lifestyle.

Now that you have the basic knowledge, let's discuss more about what it involves.

16:8 is an intermittent fasting method which involves eating cycles. For 16 hours out of 24, a person fasts. During this time calorie-free drinks are fine, but no calories or solid food. For the other 8 hours, a person is free to eat and drink.

This particular fasting method is popular due to the effort level. It offers maximum results with minimal effort.

The fasting technique may not be easy at first. It is important to know you should transition into any intermittent fasting method. Especially those with longer fasting periods like 16:8. The transitioning phase should align with each person. It will depend on how fasting makes them feel and how it fits into their lifestyle.

The cycles can repeat as often as a person wishes. It can be once or twice per week. Or, every day. It depends on the person's preference.

Most people use the 16:8 method for weight loss. It has shown more impressive results of weight loss than other popular diets. According to sources, the majority of dieters lose around 3-8% of their body weight during the fast (13).

The fasting method does not only promote weight loss. 16:8 is also believed to improve blood sugar control and boost brain function (14).

The next step is to get started. To do so, the first step is to choose when to fast and when to eat.

The majority choose to have dinner and skip breakfast the next morning. If you stop eating at 7.pm, you can then eat at 11.a.m the next day. This allows time for a late breakfast or early lunch, a snack, and dinner.

Or, some like to have their 8-hour eating window between 9.a.m and 5.p.m. This allows time for 3 healthy balanced meals. Such as a healthy breakfast, lunch, and light dinner.

The time cycles will depend on the individual and should suit your lifestyle. Making sure the times work around your routine will work best to help you sustain the fasting cycles. It is good to experiment.

Then, to maximize results you should consume nutritious and balanced foods.

Every day you should aim for healthy and hearty foods. This includes fruits, vegetables, whole grains, healthy fats, and protein.

For the vegan part of this diet, you should eat no animal products.

For the keto part of the diet, carbohydrates are to be set to a limit of around 40 grams or less per day. Thus, the list of the typical 16:8 foods are different.

For the vegan keto diet, here is a list of foods to enjoy:

- **Plant-based high protein alternatives**: tempeh, tofu, seitan
- **Low carb vegetables**: leafy greens, broccoli, cauliflower, zucchini, peppers, mushrooms, cucumber
- **High-fat dairy alternatives**: unsweetened coconut-based dairy (milks and creams), vegan cheeses, vegan butter
- **Nuts, seeds and nut butters**: pistachios, almonds, sunflower seeds, pumpkin seeds
- **Fruits**: raspberries, blackberries, avocados and other low glycemic impact berries in small quantities
- **Healthy fats/oils**: coconut oil, olive oil, MCT oil, avocado oil, macadamia oil, sesame oil

Drinking water and unsweetened teas will curb hunger and keep you hydrated.

If you are seeking meal plans to help you begin, they are in the upcoming chapters. As will be more food lists for shopping purposes. All knowledge from me to you will help you start and maintain your journey.

Do not believe everything you read for the best tips and advice for these diets. Many share incorrect knowledge due to lack of experience. It is best to follow advice like this from an educated source.

Likewise, many myths are surrounding the topic of fasting.

6

INTERMITTENT FASTING MYTHS

There are many myths to be aware of to understand what it is and is not true. Like any dieting technique, many myths are surrounding intermittent fasting. In particular, many question its ability to decrease or inhibit health conditions.

MYTH: You can eat as much as you want.

This is the number one myth many people believe is true. It is far from the truth.

Intermittent fasting is like any other diet. You should restrict calories, which means you cannot eat as much as you want.

Meals should be satisfying yet healthy. During eating windows, you should eat balanced meals. These meals should include limited carbs and saturated fats. Your meals should include plant-based proteins and healthy fats.

Overeating is counterproductive and is not the way to fast.

MYTH: Fasting for weight loss is better than other diets.

Intermittent fasting can encourage weight loss. Yet, it is not the only diet that helps a person lose weight.

Fasting is a basic dieting method. It is more of a lifestyle than a one time diet. There is no evidence to suggest that fasting is better than other dieting methods

MYTH: Fasting increases hunger.

When a person begins fasting, hunger will occur. But, over time the body adjusts due to the release of the cortisol hormone. This hormone helps control appetite and curb hunger. The release of cortisol increases during fasting.

Hunger will decrease if a person eats enough protein and healthy fats. This is because these foods digest slower and can be a source of energy for longer.

MYTH: You're going to lose weight no matter what.

Although intermittent fasting can encourage weight loss, it is not always the case. Fasting should be strict. If a person does not stick to the fasting windows or eats unhealthy meals, weight loss may not occur.

It is a common misconception for people to believe fasting is the key to weight loss success. If you eat balanced meals and exercise, weight loss will improve.

Breaking a fast with high fat or high carb foods can also inhibit weight loss results. Avoid these foods if you wish to reap the weight benefits fasting can provide.

MYTH: Fasting will slow down your metabolism.

Many people believe that metabolism will slow down because you eat less. This is incorrect.

Intermittent fasting is not about calorie restriction. Instead, it is restricting the time frame which you eat. Eating a few hours outside of your usual window will not affect the metabolic rate. You need to make sure you eat enough to avoid metabolism slowing down. Lack of food and calories can result in the metabolism slowing down.

MYTH: You cannot workout whilst fasting.

The great thing about intermittent fasting is that you can exercise. During eating windows a person can consume all the necessary foods to rebuild energy. If a person eats the right foods, this energy will be enough to sustain a workout.

Many fasters like to exercise whilst fasting as it enhances fat burning. Exercising on an empty stomach is often the best way for a person to have a successful workout.

MYTH: Fasting is better than snacking for weight loss.

It is important to know that intermittent fasting and snacking are different. Neither is better for weight loss than the other. Fasting is healthier and more sustainable. But, each involves decreasing calorie intake which results in weight loss.

Calorie deficit is the key to success for weight loss. No matter if you are eating fewer meals or less food, both involve a calorie deficit. This means both can result in weight loss.

MYTH: You should eat a big meal when you break your fast.

Overeating when breaking a fast can cause more damage than you think. When you break your fast it should not involve high carbohydrate foods. This is because it can result in fatigue and a spike in blood sugar.

A small meal is better for breaking a fast. It is best to eat your biggest meal before beginning a fast.

MYTH: You will be very fit and healthy from fasting.

Like with any diet, a person should have a healthy lifestyle to maximize results. Fasting alone will not result in a fit and healthy physique and body.

There is no magic dieting method. Thus, a person should have a healthy lifestyle whilst fasting to achieve the best results.

MYTH: Everyone gets the same results.

All intermittent fasting methods offer different results. The same goes for people. Each person will achieve different results. There is no definition for which method and type of person will achieve the best results.

MYTH: It is good because our bodies cannot digest food overnight.

It is good for your body to not be full during sleep. This is because of a lack of movement means digestion will be slower. But, your digestive system does still work overnight. It works no matter the time of day. When a person eats, that food begins to digest. If you eat in the middle of the night, your body will digest it.

It's a matter of allowing your body a significant time to focus on metabolic processes. Whether that is 12 or 18 hours between meals, digestion always happens.

MYTH: Skipping breakfast makes you fat.

Most believe that breakfast is the most important meal of the day. People say that it kicks your metabolism.

Your metabolism is always working to digest food. Your body is not aware if you are eating breakfast or dinner. When a person eats, metabolism will kickstart.

Studies show that there is no difference in weight when a person skips breakfast or not.

7

HOW TO INTERMITTENT FAST

Intermittent fasting methods are all different and involve their own individual rules. All involve their own fasting and eating windows. Some involve strict calorie control. Others involve regular eating with cycles of fasting. Fasting windows can vary depending on the method and the person.

More on how to fast is in the '5 Types of Intermittent Fasting' chapter.

When you know how to fast for your chosen method, it is time to work out a schedule.

Working Out A Schedule

Your schedule should align with your lifestyle. It will also depend on the chosen method of intermittent fasting.

Let us make a scenario. Let's say you choose the 16:8 method. Your job does not coincide with the 16-hour fast window. You will have to prioritize. If you start work early and need to have breakfast at home, then begin your fast early.

Your schedule should revolve around your lifestyle and priorities. Each week may involve a different fasting schedule because of that. If so, you should plan ahead to ensure you successfully fast to maximize results.

If one week you cannot fast, then don't. The good thing about intermittent fasting is that you can start and stop when you need to.

But, starting and stopping often will not offer maximum results.

Once your schedule is final, the next step is to put a plan into place. This involves everything from meal planning to exercising.

Putting A Plan In Place

Planning your fasting routine is a great success tool. Once you've chosen your fasting method and found a schedule that fits, a plan will allow it all to work together.

Like any dieting technique, meal and exercise plans help. They encourage you to stay on track.

Like scheduling, planning is also specific to the fasting method you choose. In general, there are no specific meal plans for intermittent fasting. Instead, you should eat nutritious balanced meals. Avoid snacking or overeating to achieve the best results.

It is safe to exercise whilst fasting. Whether that be after eating or during the fast. Some like to exercise on an empty stomach. Others like to exercise after eating. Either plan is fine and safe. It depends on the person.

Exercising alongside fasting is also very beneficial. It can increase weight loss and improves the mental attitude towards fasting.

Find more on specific meal plans for intermittent fasting and the vegan keto diet in the following chapter.

Staying On Track

With most diets, people need encouragement. A buddy or partner to influence you is key for staying on track. Whilst most associate a diet buddy to be human, nowadays that buddy can be your smartphone.

All smartphones can download apps. Nowadays there is an app for everything. There are even intermittent fasting apps. These work to guide you through your fasting cycles. You can use them as a fasting tracker.

The most popular app on the market is Zero. It is an intuitive fasting tracker with all the essential fasting tools. See it as your fasting coach. Along the way, the app rewards you with badges to celebrate milestones.

Zero includes a tracker as its number one tool. Then, there are tools and statistics to teach you about intermittent fasting. There are also premium features including videos and articles to offer more insight. Zero also offers journaling for you to write notes to look back on. Everything is an act of encouragement and guidance.

An app is a good and easy way to keep up to date with your new fasting window. Instead of having to remember when to fast and break the fast each day, this will do it for you. It will even send you notifications to remind you to start and stop eating.

There are other alternative intermittent fasting apps if you are keen to try others. This includes Fastient, Body-Fast, and Vora. After Zero, Fastient is the top trending for note-taking. So if you like to journal to look back on progress, this is your app.

If you would like help with meal planning, BodyFast is most popular for that. It offers many different meal plans as well as coaching.

Vora offers a community that you can gain extra

support from. If you like having human interaction during a diet or fasting routine, Vora is the answer.

Search your application store to see the top trending and best reviews. All offer different essential tools.

Or, many Facebook groups can provide support and motivation for intermittent fasting. You can join today our Facebook group dedicated to Intermittent Fasting, you will surely be encouraged.

As well as your own journey, you may be wondering more about the real results of intermittent fasting. In every diet journey, weight loss is the main goal. Intermittent fasting has proven to offer amazing weight loss benefits.

8

INTERMITTENT FASTING FOR
WEIGHT LOSS

I ntermittent fasting is an effective way to lose weight. Many studies conclude that intermittent fasting can offer weight loss to every participant.

First, it can help you eat fewer calories and less food in general. Restricting how much you eat is a natural and effective way to lose weight.

According to studies, intermittent fasting may reduce body weight by up to 8%. The study also saw a decrease in body fat by up to 16% over 3 to 12 weeks (15).

Intermittent fasting can also kick start fat-burning hormones. This hormone is norepinephrine, which excels in metabolic rates and increases fat burning (16). The hormone works by speeding up energy expenditure. The quicker release of energy allows your body to burn glucose as well as fat. When the body runs out of glucose, it turns to fat for fuel. This is the ketosis process, which is a huge benefit of intermittent fasting (17).

When paired with a ketogenic diet, intermittent fasting can speed up ketosis. Which amplifies weight loss. Both diet methods promote ketosis. Thus, the two together excel weight loss further.

Intermittent fasting also shows positive results for gaining leaner muscles (18). This is due to calorie restriction. Body composition improvements are a huge benefit of fasting.

Yet to achieve the best results, you need to put in as much work as the fast does. To lose the most weight and achieve your goals, you must maintain a healthy lifestyle. Without exercise and healthy eating, the results will be less effective.

As well as weight loss, intermittent fasting offers many other real results.

9

INTERMITTENT FASTING RESULTS

I ntermittent fasting has been an interesting area of study for many years. Besides weight loss, it promotes other health benefits. This includes better heart health and inhibiting certain cancers. All have shown real results. Thus, concluding that intermittent fasting does work.

Science proves that intermittent fasting can prevent particular diseases and conditions. For example, a 2018 study found that the 16:8 method can reduce blood pressure in obese adults (19). In the study, obese individuals found that the 8-hour fasting window saw a drop in blood pressure. Then, when breaking the fast the blood pressure did increase but not as much as before fasting. Suggesting that the fast encourages a decrease in blood pressure.

Fasting helps reduce blood pressure in obese individuals better than healthy weight individuals. This is due to obesity causing a spike in blood pressure. Thus, it is easier to decrease.

Many reports are concluding that intermittent fasting

can also help diabetic patients. In particular, by decreasing glucose and insulin levels.

In a study, participants were fasting for 8 hours. During the fasting window, people saw a 3 to 6% decrease in glucose levels. In the same study, they saw a decrease in insulin by up to 57% (20). These two signal positive benefits for type 2 diabetic patients. As they deal with an imbalance in glucose and insulin. Balancing these levels during fasting is an ideal way to improve them when eating. It prevents a dramatic decrease or increase occurring when eating. This is helpful to manage diabetes.

Much research attempts to discover how and why exercising is good during fasting.

10

INTERMITTENT FASTING & WORKING OUT

Studies show that exercising whilst fasting burns more off leftover glycogen (21). Glycogen is glucose. When glycogen runs out, fat is then the substitute as an energy source. Thus suggesting that exercising whilst fasting burns fat better than exercising after eating.

You replace your glucose when eating. This means that the energy used during a workout is the energy from the glucose in the food.

Working out whilst fasting is dependent on the individual. Some may prefer to work out before beginning the fast. This is because people like to work off their food and feel they have the most energy. But, some prefer to work out on an empty stomach. Depending on the person, this preference will change.

There is not enough evidence to state if exercising whilst fasting burns more fat. Yet, it can burn off excess fat when the body runs out of glycogen. This suggests fasting does offer great fat-burning benefits.

Another preference is the type of workout a person wishes to do whilst fasting. If a person does choose to exercise whilst fasting, it can range from HIIT to muscle gaining. Again, this depends on preference and current energy levels. Strength works out and requires more energy and carbohydrates. Whilst high-intensity interval training (HIIT) requires less carbohydrates and energy.

Depending on your preferred time and type of workout, a person should eat the right foods to fuel the energy. Without energy, your body will feel tired and overworked. Always ensure you do not workout if your body cannot manage it. Fasting can lead to fatigue, which can worsen with exercise.

Regardless of time or type of exercise, you should always hydrate yourself. Drinking plenty of water is beneficial in many ways during fasting. It can curb cravings and control appetite. Also, hydration can lead to better workouts and less fatigue. Drinking more water than usual whilst fasting is common. And, also a good thing to keep up to reduce tiredness and fatigue.

A downside to exercising whilst fasting is that the body may become too tired. Fatigue is a common side effect of fasting. Working out on a small amount of remaining energy may overwork your body. Your body depletes itself of energy, which could end up slowing your metabolism.

A workout should be dependent on your energy levels at the time. Advice to take is to not exercise if you already feel tired.

11

DOES INTERMITTENT FASTING WORK WITHOUT EXERCISE?

I ntermittent fasting is not a magic pill. It cannot offer the best results without exercise.

Intermittent fasting may still offer weight loss benefits. Even without exercise, it can improve results. For example, if your goal is to burn fat then exercise can excel that. Exercising alongside fasting can increase results and help you achieve your goal quicker (22).

Intermittent fasting is often a method for achieving leaner muscles. This is due to the ketosis process encouraging your body to burn fat. Burning fat will result in leaner muscles. Without exercise, the body can lose fat as much as it can muscle. Thus, muscle mass may deteriorate without the right exercise.

Yet, intermittent fasting can still work without exercise for other health benefits. This is because the other health benefits do not need exercise to maximize results.

For example, intermittent fasting can reduce blood sugar levels. It can also improve blood pressure and triglycerides (23). These health benefits do not need exercise to occur.

Some existing health conditions may need to avoid exercise. Thus, does need exercise for intermittent fasting to take effect.

There is no right or wrong answer to this. It depends on what a person is using fasting for to say whether exercise is necessary. If a person is seeking weight loss then exercise can improve results. For other health benefits, fasting does not need exercise to maximize results.

12

AUTOPHAGY & FASTING

Autophagy is an action in which the body clears out damaged cells. It is a natural regulatory process where a cell removes dysfunctional components. A cell would work to remove organelles, proteins, and cell membranes that it no longer needs. The part of the cell that works to remove the dysfunctional components is in the lysosomes. The unhealthy old proteins go to the lysosomes to die (24).

After some time, cells divide so much that they die. This process is essential for maintaining good health.

This cycle makes room for newer and healthier cells. The literal meaning of autophagy is "self-eating". The words are Greek. Auto means self and phagy means eating.

Christian de Duve found autophagy in 1963. But the understanding of the process was due to the discovery of how it is beneficial for the body. This research was complete in 2016 by Japanese biologist Yoshinori Ohsumi. The studies found that autophagy can prevent illnesses due to the healthy cycle of new cells (25). The cells that die during autophagy are ones that could cause illnesses. Thus, the removal process allows room for new cells. It also decreases the chance of developing illnesses.

Autophagy can benefit regulatory inflammatory and infectious diseases (26). It can help with certain forms of cancer and work as a treatment method, like chemotherapy. The studies reveal it can also reduce neurodegenerative diseases. Such as Parkinson's and Alzheimer's disease. Autophagy also has the potential to inhibit metabolic diseases and autoimmune diseases. Recent research shows how it may also benefit depression and mental disorders (27).

But, not everyone can achieve autophagy. Your past or current health will state if it's safe to achieve autophagy.

Nutrient deprivation is the key activator for autophagy (28). This often occurs during fasting. Thus, fasting is the number one way to activate autophagy.

When the body eats insulin increases and glucagon decreases. The opposite occurs when the body doesn't eat. During periods of not eating, insulin decreases, and glucagon increases. Autophagy needs glucagon to activate. Thus, verifying that fasting stimulates autophagy. Then, autophagy stops when a person eats as it decreases glucagon.

More research needs to verify the exact timing the body needs to fast for to stimulate autophagy. Yet, scientists have found that autophagy begins after 18 hours of fasting. One study found this to be the case in the majority of participants. The same study found that peak results occur after 48 hours (29).

There are five sequential steps for the autophagy process. It begins with the initiation of autophagy. This involves a lack of food and nutrients. Nutrient deprivation triggers autophagy. Then, elongation and maturation occurs. This is where the proteins in the cells fuse into the lysosome. Here is where the degradation of the dysfunctional components occurs. These components die and make room for new components.

There are only a few definite ways to see if your body is going through autophagy. This includes having a low blood glucose level. Low blood glucose indicates the body is going through the ketosis process (30). This is the beginning of autophagy.

Low insulin levels can also state autophagy. Fasting and low carb diets all encourage low insulin levels. Both of these diets stimulate autophagy.

Autophagy is beneficial for weight loss. Thus, indicators of successful autophagy include weight loss, reduced appetite, and muscle loss. Lack of food induces the autophagy process as much as it helps a person eat less.

When a person is trying to achieve peak autophagy is important to hydrate the body. This helps with a total body cleanse. You can infuse the water with fruits if you wish to. It is also essential to eat nutrient-dense meals during eating windows. This will replace the lost nutrients during the fast and autophagy process.

Whether a person should try and achieve autophagy will depend on their health. You should check your past or current health conditions with a doctor to see if it is safe. Autophagy requires a certain extent of fasting, which may not be safe for everyone.

Fasting in general is also not recommended for underweight people. Neither is it safe for pregnant people, children, and the very elderly.

Like autophagy, intermittent fasting is not for everyone.

13

INTERMITTENT FASTING SIDE EFFECTS

Intermittent fasting is not for everyone, like most dieting techniques. With all fasting methods come a few side effects and risks that you should be aware of. For the most part, intermittent fasting has very few risks and is more often than not, safe.

Most side effects are temporary. But, if side effects are consistent, then a person should stop fasting. Then, if necessary you should see a doctor to prevent any health complications.

Hunger is the main side effect of intermittent fasting due to lack of food. The time takes time to adjust to a lack of food. If a person usually eats late at night or first thing in the morning, they will notice this. Hunger during fasting will reduce after a few weeks of doing it. The body adjusts to the new cycle of eating and not eating within a few weeks.

There are other side effects to be cautious of:

- Weakness

- Fatigue
- Slow reactions
- Irritability
- Dehydration

With hunger being a main side effect, many people need encouragement to sustain the fast. Managing to stay on track and succeed in fasting will conclude with great results. Once your body passes the mild side effects, you can be on track and fast to your fullest potential.

There are many ways to boost results with intermittent fasting. Depending on which method you choose, here are the top tips for excelling your results:

- Avoid sugars and grains. Instead of sugary foods and grains, eat natural foods low in sugar. This includes fruits, vegetables, legumes, whole grains, lean proteins, and healthy fats.
- Avoid snacking by pre-occupying your mind. Snacking is best to avoid. Try and be active during periods you feel you want a snack to build muscle tone and keep your mind active.
- Start with an easy intermittent fasting method. Test out the simple and less restrictive fasting methods first. This will allow your body time to ease into the longer fasts.
- Avoid eating at night time. The digestive system has to work extra hard to burn food overnight whilst it's resting. Try to avoid eating after 8.p.m to let your gut rest and not overwork.

Due to food restrictions, fasting can have a negative effect on certain individuals. There are a few people/medical conditions which should avoid intermittent fasting. Or fasting in general. Below is a list of people that should avoid fasting or seek advice before starting.

Diabetic patients

Diabetic patients are of the majority that need to consult a doctor before fasting. Due to the issue with insulin fluctuation, fasting may cause more damage. Fasting can raise blood glucose, which is detrimental for diabetics.

Fasting has proven to have a positive effect on insulin resistance. But a person should still check their insulin before fasting. This is to check if you are safe to fast, discuss with your doctor before committing to a fast. You may find the mild side effects come into effect but are worse.

Anyone with a current or past eating disorder

Fasting is often a weight-loss tool and for the majority, it will cause weight loss. Weight loss occurs more so with calorie restriction and long fasts. Anyone with a current or past eating disorder may notice severe weight gain or loss when fasting.

Fasting increases cortisol, the hunger hormone (31). Thus, for those who have an issue with weight control may struggle. Fasting is detrimental for anyone with existing strict eating habits. Or, for those who are underweight. Anyone underweight should avoid fasting as it can cause weight to decline further. This can result in anorexia or bulimia.

Fasting is for good intentions. Never use fasting as a primary weight loss tool if you are suspect to eating disorders. It can have a detrimental impact on your health and cause severe consequences.

Low blood pressure

Fasting has shown to lower blood pressure. Thus, those who already have low blood pressure should avoid fasting. It may cause blood pressure to drop to a dangerous level and result in severe consequences.

Underweight individuals

Anyone who has a history of anorexia or being underweight should avoid fasting. As should those who are currently underweight.

Fastings number one benefit is weight loss. Thus, anyone underweight will cause damage to their health.

Women trying to get pregnant/are pregnant or breastfeeding

Reports have shown that fasting for too long can cause ovulation to slow down. Thus, in some cases, it may make conceiving difficult. Fasting also causes weight loss which can also make trying to get pregnant difficult. It is important to take all necessary precautions if you are trying to conceive.

Scientists suggest women who are breastfeeding need extra calories daily. This is to ensure a woman can provide enough healthy breast milk. Women also need all vitamins during breastfeeding, especially B12. Fasting can cause nutrient deficiencies. Again, this is something to take precaution of if you are breastfeeding.

Those who fast for religious reasons are often exempt from the practice.

Women with current or past amenorrhea

Amenorrhea is the absence of menstruation. It is often due to dramatic weight loss or menstrual conditions. Sometimes it can be due to nutritional deficiencies. Fasting can sometimes result in deficiencies and weight loss. This makes it common for amenorrhea patients to avoid fasting.

Weight loss is the main benefit of fasting. Thus, those with current or past amenorrhea should avoid fasting. It can cause further weight loss which can cause the condition to worsen.

Fasting a few times a month will not cause amenorrhea or significant weight loss. Not so much that the weight loss will be damaging to the body.

Most of those recommended to avoid intermittent fasting seem to be women. The reason being because research suggests the fasting methods may not be as effective on women as it is on men. Also, fasting techniques have a big influence on hormone changes.

Due to the change in hormones, intermittent fasting can pose dangers for females. More so than men. For these reasons, women should be particularly cautious when fasting.

14

INTERMITTENT FASTING FOR MEN

I ntermittent fasting offers more benefits than risks for men. In general, there are fewer risks for men. The main issue a man may notice whilst fasting is fatigue, which is due to lack of food. Over time, mild side effects like fatigue will ease off as the body adjusts to the fasting cycle.

Once the body adjusts, intermittent fasting leaves people feeling energized. In particular, this can encourage people to exercise more.

The International Society of Sports Nutrition reports that fasting can improve body composition (32). Whilst this can be beneficial for both men and women, it can be encouraging for men. Males tend to exercise to gain muscle mass. In general, men aim to be leaner with increased muscle mass. This is easier to achieve with fasting due to the change in diet.

Fasting allows the body to detox and balance out fat and muscle mass. Reports show that intermittent fasting can be better than a regular diet for muscle gain. The cycles encourage people to eat better balanced meals. This should involve protein, healthy fats, and limited carbohydrates. This is easy to sustain for any lifestyle.

Whilst fasting, it is better to eat nutritious meals to avoid deficiencies. That is the benefit of the vegan keto diet. You will be limiting carbohydrate intake whilst eating plant-based meals. Your diet will already be full of low carb, high plant-based foods. This makes it easier and natural to eat balanced meals.

If you are seeking body improvements, some fasting methods are better than others. For example, 16:8 is easier to maintain and will allow your body the nutrients it needs to gain muscle and lose fat. Whereas alternate day fasting or 5:2 are less sustainable. But, they will still encourage improvements. This is because 16:8 is more of a lifestyle than a diet. Thus, it will feel natural and help a person eat the right foods.

The intermittent fasting method a person chooses will depend on goals and lifestyle.

15

INTERMITTENT FASTING FOR WOMEN

I ntermittent fasting reacts to the female body in a different way to the male body. The main cause of this is due to hormonal changes.

Many studies display that intermittent fasting may not be as beneficial for women as it is men. The main complications are with heart health and menstruation (33). Reference

This research shows that blood sugar control is more difficult for women than men. A study saw that women who fasted for over 3 weeks had difficulty with controlling blood sugar. In the same study, men had no difficulty.

The women in the study saw an impairment with glucose from food after the 3 week fasting period (34). This meant that glucose response was slow after each meal. Which concludes women may suffer from glucose intolerance during fasting. This can result in irregular blood sugar levels.

Female bodies are sensitive to calorie restrictions. More so than men. This is due to the hormone changes that come with a lack of food and certain nutrients.

There are many reports of women having difficulties with natural menstruation whilst fasting (35). Calorie restrictions can cause weight loss. Weight loss is a common cause of menstruation issues like amenorrhea. Disruption to the menstrual cycle can make it difficult for a woman to become pregnant.

Calorie restriction can slow down the release of gonadotropin-releasing hormone (GnRH). This is a hormone that helps release two more reproductive hormones. Which are the luteinizing hormone (LH) and the follicle-stimulating hormone (FSH). Research has shown that the decrease of certain hormones can cause ovaries to shrink (36). If this happens, it can be common for women to have less or missed periods. Reproductive hormones help the ovaries communicate. Without them, a woman may experience irregular menstrual cycles or infertility. The lack of these hormones can also cause poor bone health.

There are more complications for women than men, yet there are also many health benefits. We cover the complications so that you are aware and can take the necessary precautions.

16

PROS AND CONS OF INTERMITTENT FASTING

L ike all diets, there are positives and negatives. Intermittent fasting offers many health benefits. Yet, there are a few cons to be aware of. There are some things to consider before starting intermittent fasting. Here are the most common pros and cons people need to weigh up.

Pros

Helps with weight loss

The number one benefit of intermittent fasting is weight loss. When fasting alongside exercise, results can be greater. How much effort a person contributes to fasting will impact their results.

Has anti-inflammatory benefits

Fasting can offer amazing anti-inflammatory benefits. These benefits can be for illnesses, the gut, skin, and much more. Fasting helps with inflammation due to a reduction in cells that cause inflammation. These are cells found in the blood, known as monocytes.

Improves gut and heart health

Intermittent fasting gives your gut and heart a break from working. In particular, fasting gives your digestive system a break. Fasting allows your body to adhere to its circadian rhythm. It helps your body know when to enter the best metabolic state. This due to nutrient availability. It helps your body know to burn fats instead of sugars. This is very beneficial for gut health as much as it is for weight loss.

For heart health, fasting improves blood pressure and sugar levels. It does this due to calorie control and better eating patterns.

Reduces the risk of disease and illness

There is much evidence to prove how fasting can reduce the risk of diseases. Fasting can reduce the risk of inflammation conditions. It can also reduce or inhibit heart conditions. There are a variety of ways in which intermittent fasting can reduce the risk of illnesses.

Beneficial for diabetic patients

Intermittent fasting methods can also improve insulin sensitivity. Which is essential for type 2 diabetes patients. It also helps the body manage glucose from the foods you eat. Some research even suggests that fasting can prevent diabetes. This is due to its ability to balance glucose and insulin.

Aids better digestion

Intermittent fasting allows the digestive system a break. A break can help break down foods quicker and easier. During the first few weeks of fasting, the digestive system may struggle. This may be due to the change in eating patterns. But, with time the digestive system can improve and have a healthier cycle for breaking down food.

Cons

Can interfere with social eating

If you get an invite to a social event during a fasting period, this may be an issue. It is important to not be too strict with fasting. Allow yourself to have time off when you feel it is necessary.

May induce low energy and productivity

Lack of essential nutrients may cause the body to feel low on energy. Fatigue is common. Especially during the first few fast cycles. Energy is easy to replace with drinks such as water and coffee. Replenish your hunger with liquid. This will prevent low energy and breaking your fast early.

Can cause people to overeat during eating windows

During the first few weeks, it is common for people to feel hungrier than usual. This can sometimes cause people to overeat when breaking a fast. Overeating will not benefit your body and can inhibit you from achieving results.

May cause digestion issues

The digestive system may take a while to adjust to the new eating pattern. It is important to ease yourself back into eating after a fasting period. This is to prevent blockage. Too much food may also cause the digestive system to go into overload and have to overwork. It is better to break a fast with a small nutritious meal.

Can cause stress

As the body may become more tired than usual, the mind may experience more stress. Stress is often due to fatigue and is common during the first few fasts.

People may experience mild side effects

For most people, it can take time for the body to adjust to intermittent fasting. The body may experience fatigue and hunger which can also induce irritability. This can continue until the body adjusts. It is common to experience hunger during the first few fasts. To avoid extreme hunger and fatigue, it is important to keep the body hydrated. It is fine to drink calorie-free drinks when fasting. Water, black tea, and coffee will decrease hunger and control appetite.

The cons of intermittent fasting can be under control with the right practice. Most cons are a cause of the mild side effects that occur during the first few weeks of fasting. To prevent and control this, follow the above advice.

All bodies are different and adjust to intermittent fasting methods in different ways. Give your body time to adjust. Do not continue with fasting if you experience severe side effects or complications.

FAQ

How much weight can you lose in a month with intermittent fasting?

The amount of weight a person can lose will depend on a variety of factors. Such as current weight, diet, lifestyle and exercise routine. Then, how much effort you put into the fasting method will dictate how much weight a person can lose. For example, if you do not abide by the dietary restrictions 100%, the results may not be as great.

Studies show how a person can lose between 3 and 8 percent of their body weight after 3 weeks, up to 24 weeks (37). The majority of participants lost an average of 0.55 pounds per week.

Can I drink liquid during the fast?

Yes, you can drink liquid during the fast. The drinks must be calorie-free which includes water, black tea, and black coffee.

Can I take supplements whilst fasting?

Most studies suggest that supplements are fine to take during fasting. They are best to consume when the fast stops, during the eating period. It is often encouraged to take supplements for long fasting methods. Or, if you choose to fast as a lifestyle, you should take supplements too. This is because some people may experience nutritional deficiencies.

How long does it take to see results?

Most reports say that it will take several weeks to see significant results. Sometimes reports state it can take up to 10 weeks. This can be due to individuals only fasting one or two days per week. Additionally, as there are many methods of intermittent fasting, results vary.

Results will depend on the individual and their chosen fasting method.

Why am I gaining weight with intermittent fasting?

When a person restricts their calories, weight will often be a result of that. But, if a person overeats during the eating window, then it is more than likely that the person will gain weight.

During eating windows you should keep meals balanced, avoid overeating, and unnecessary snacking.

Can I do intermittent fasting everyday?

It is safe to intermittent fasting everyday if you choose certain methods, such as 16:8. After a few weeks of fasting, your body will adjust. It will feel natural for your body to control appetite better at certain times of the day.

Some methods of intermittent fasting are not safe to do daily, such as alternate day methods. It is not safe to fast for days on end. The safest method is time-restricted eating such as 16:8.

What breaks an intermittent fast?

Anything that contains calories will break an intermittent fast. This can be a calorie drink or any food.

When you do break the fast, a small low carbohydrate meal is best to prevent your blood sugar from spiking.

Can I exercise during fasting?

It is safe to exercise whilst fasting, even if choosing the extended 24 hour fast. As long as your body has enough energy and hydration, it will cope if you exercise often.

Fasted cardiovascular exercise linked with excelled fat burning. It is a good technique to use if your goal is to burn fat.

Does intermittent fasting slow down metabolism?

Intermittent fasting has shown to actually increase the metabolic rate. During short-term intermittent fasting, studies show an increase in metabolism for all participants.

Metabolism can slow down if the fast is longer than 3

days, which it isn't. But, religious fasting can be for longer than this period and if so, metabolism can slow down here.

To make your intermittent fasting journey successful there are a few things we can suggest. Keeping track of your routine with a journal can help you see progress. It can also encourage you to make a habit or lifestyle of fasting.

It also helps to be mindful when fasting. Take time to exercise and energize your body to help you stay active and on track with the food cycles. This can prevent weight gain and control your food consumption.

Make your intermittent fasting routine personal to you. This will help you be active and maintain fasting as a life-style. It offers so many health benefits that can be benefi-cial for a lifetime. If you are safe to fast, it is definitely worth partaking in fasting.

PART II

VEGAN DIET 101

"Cows scream louder than carrots."

*— **Alan Watts***

1

WHAT IS VEGANISM?

Veganism practices abstaining from the use, and consumption of animal products. It rejects the commodification of animals. Veganism excludes all exploitation, and cruelty of animal products. This includes food as well as clothing, and any other purposes.

The vegan diet consumes plant products as a substitute for animal products. Meat, dairy, eggs, and other animal substances are not prohibited on the vegan diet.

Scientists suggest that almost 8% of the worldwide population is now practicing veganism.

More people have decided to become vegan due to other reasons than their health. Veganism is also ethical, and environmental. When a vegan diet is 100% abided by and successful, there are many health benefits a person can reap. It can help with weight loss, blood sugar control, and much more.

Veganism is in some ways a more extreme version of vegetarianism. There is a similarity due to the exclusion of meat. Yet, veganism excludes both the consumption and use of all animal products.

Plant-based diets date back as far as 500BCE in the writings of the Greek philosopher, Pythagoras of Samos. Yet, there was not an exact definition. Nor was their research to conclude that veganism can offer health benefits.

Veganism was better defined, understood, and coined in 1944 by Donald Watson. The vegan diet is now known as a modern-day diet amongst those who share the same views. It was almost coined the "non-dairy vegetarian" diet by Donald Watson, and peers. But, they felt the definition did not cover the exclusion of all animal products. That is when the term veganism came around.

The vegan diet has grown in popularity in more recent years. This is due to better scientific research, and more plant-based food options. With many sustainable plant-based foods on the market, it is now easier than ever to manage a vegan diet.

Since 2016, the vegan population has more than doubled. It has increased from 276,000 vegans worldwide in 2016 to over 600,000 in 2019.

The vegan diet is one that consumes only plant-based products. This includes vegetables, grains, nuts, fruits, and any other food made from plants.

This diet should not get confused with vegetarianism. Vegetarians allow the consumption of some animal products. For example, they consume dairy and eggs.

Whereas, veganism practices the exclusion of animal product consumption, and use. Thus, the vegan diet includes no meat, dairy, or eggs. Other products contain animal products. This includes certain sauces, honey, candy, beers, and wines.

The vegan diet is now seen as a way of living. There are many reasons for people consuming the vegan diet. It is not consumed for personal health benefits. But, to also improve the environment and ethics.

2

WHAT FOODS TO EAT, AND AVOID ON
THE VEGAN DIET

I t is easy to understand that the vegan diet eliminates all animal products. But, you may wonder exactly what you should eat in the replacement of those animal products. Also how to sustain it, and make it work for you.

With the right balanced foods, it is easy to achieve a healthy vegan diet. It is as simple as finding what foods you like. Ensuring you eat nutritious, dense foods will help you maximize results, and benefits. It will also help inhibit any nutrient deficiencies. As well as reducing any mild side effects, such as fatigue. Preventing these may help you sustain the vegan diet long term.

For a healthy, and successful diet you should start with finding food substitutions. This will help understand what to base your meals around.

Substitutes for meat

Plant-based products are more popular than ever as meat substitutes. This includes tofu, tempeh, and seitan. More and more brands are creating their own plant-based substitutes. Many are now a great source of protein which acts as a great replacement.

Another great meat substitute is legumes and beans. It is simple to replace meat or other animal produce in your meals with these. Legumes and beans are a popular vegan choice. Beans, lentils, and peas are all vegan, and great sources of nutrients, and also protein.

Substitutes for dairy

There are even more substitutes for dairy than for meat. For milk, you can choose from a variety of soy-based or nuts milk. This includes soya, almond, coconut, oat, rice, hazelnut, and cashew milk.

There are many vegan products to replace dairy products. All of which are soy or nut-based products. There are many vegan kinds of cheese, milk, and creams on the market.

Finding the right substitutes to replace animal products is key. From there you can begin to discover new foods and your favorite meals. Then, it will feel more of a lifestyle to be vegan. Eating the right foods will help you reap the health benefits veganism offers. Below is a list of the healthy, and nutrient-dense foods to consume whilst being on the vegan diet.

- **The meat substitutes**: all foods mentioned above. This includes tofu, tempeh, seitan, legumes, pulses, and beans.
- **The dairy substitutes**: all non-dairy alternatives shared above are vegan. Non-dairy milk, yogurts, cheese, creams, and more are

perfect. Most contain similar fat and protein content to natural dairy products. If you worry about lacking in calcium, there is a good alternative. There are many calcium-fortified plant milk and yogurts in supermarkets. They help increase your calcium intake and provide you with a good source of vitamin D, and B12.

- **Algae**: Algae is a great alternative source of protein. Vegans cannot consume whey protein. Which is what many meat-eaters use to increase their protein intake. So, the alga is an ideal source of plant protein. It also contains an impressive amount of amino acids. You can add algae to juices, smoothies, and salads.

- **Whole grains**: complex carbs are a great addition to any diet. Whole grains are good for vegans. They offer many essential nutrients, that they may be deficient in. This includes fiber, iron, vitamin B's, and minerals. Spelled, cereals, and quinoa are great options as they contain the most nutrients in a small serving. Whole grains are healthier than white grains. This is because they hold more key nutrients such as complex carbs, proteins, and fibers.

- **Fruits, and vegetables**: all fruits and vegetables are fine on the vegan diet. They are a great way to increase your nutrient intake. The best advice is to consume 5 fruits or vegetables per day.

- **Nutritional yeast**: this particular yeast is very popular amongst vegans. This is due to the lack of vitamin B in the diet. Nutritional yeast adds protein, and flavor to any vegan dish. It also has many health benefits. Including reducing cholesterol, improving immunity, and holds powerful antioxidants (38). You can use it by sprinkling over food and stirring into sauces, and soups to add flavor, and thicken them.

- **Nut, seeds, and nut butter**: research suggests it is best to consume unroasted nuts and seeds. This is so that you get the essential nutrients they contain. Nuts and seeds are high in many key nutrients and vitamins. The nutrients include protein and fiber. Then, there are many vitamins. This includes iron, selenium, magnesium, zinc, and vitamin E. Nuts, and seeds are good to top your meals with. They add flavor, nutrients, and healthy fats. Hemp, chia, sesame, and flax seeds are a great source of protein.

- **Fermented plant foods**: fermented foods improve mineral absorption. Plant-based fermented foods work in the same way non-vegan ones do. They contain probiotics which are great for improving gut health, and digestion (39). These foods include miso, sauerkraut, natto, kimchi, and kombucha. Add these to the sides of your meals for better mineral absorption.

Eating all the above foods will help you consume all essential nutrients. Which your body needs to stay healthy, and function well. They are easy to incorporate into all meals of the day. Keeping up nutrient-dense meals will maximize health benefits. It will also help you sustain the diet long term.

Foods To Avoid On The Vegan Diet

As well as foods to enjoy, they are a few you should be aware that you should avoid.

It's obvious that animal products are not okay on the vegan diet. Yet, there are a few foods you may be unaware that are not allowed on the vegan diet, those include:

- **All animal meat**: this includes meat, poultry, fish, and seafood. Although some non-meat eating diets allow fish, and seafood, the vegan diet does not.
- **Dairy**: all dairy products are not okay on the vegan diet. This includes milk, cream, cheese, yogurt, butter, and ice cream.
- **Eggs**: eggs are a food that comes from an animal. Thus, it is not okay to eat eggs on a vegan diet. All eggs are non-vegan such as duck, chicken, quail, fish, and ostrich eggs.
- **Bee products**: products from bees are animal produce. This includes honey, bee pollen, and royal jelly. Bee products are often added to candy, such as sweets, and ice creams, to add flavor.
- **Animal-based ingredients**: there are more animal-based ingredients to be aware of. This includes whey, lactose, egg white, gelatine, fish-derived omega-3 fatty acids, isinglass, shellac, carmine, animal-derived vitamin D3, and L-cysteine. These ingredients are often in alcoholic beverages, candy, and chocolate. Always check your food packaging labels to check for these ingredients. All products will be

on the label as vegan if free from all animal products.

3

VEGAN FOOD DIET PLAN

A ll vegan dieters like to choose their meals depending on preference. It is difficult to suggest a full meal plan because of this. Yet, there is some brief guidance to suggest to help you get started with the vegan diet.

Nutritional planning is key, and ideal for everyone. Ensuring you are eating balanced meals will help you achieve the essential nutrients. Which, many vegans can be low in.

You can begin with meal planning when you find your favorite plant-based foods.

Each meal should contain essential nutrients. This includes protein, fiber, carbohydrates, and minerals.

A healthy balanced meal could include a variety of nutrients. Such as whole grains, fiber, fruits, vegetables, and plant-based proteins.

For breakfast, it does not need to include all these food groups. So, oatmeal, pancakes, and cereals are a good whole grain and high fiber option. Fruits are good to put on top.

Then for savory options, plant-based proteins, and vegetables are perfect. Tofu scramble is a great substitute for scrambled eggs. With that, you could add roasted or fresh vegetables to achieve your 5 a day.

Both options are a great source of essential nutrients and energy. They are both nutritious, and well balanced. You could change them each day to change between sweet, and savory.

For lunch, whole grains or plant-based proteins should be in equal amounts. Then vegetables and fermented foods are good to add to the side or on top. An example is a couscous with chickpeas, topped with spinach, and kimchi.

Dinner can be like lunch. But, if you have not consumed a lot of protein that day, you could make up for it here. A plentiful dinner should provide all essential nutrients. A good example is a sweet potato with beans, salad, and avocado. Nuts or seeds of choice are a good addition.

Snacks are down to personal preference. The best options are nuts, seeds, fruits, and drinks. Water, teas, and juices are a good option for drinks to control hunger.

4

THE BENEFITS OF THE VEGAN DIET

There are more benefits to a vegan diet than most may assume. Many associate vegan dieting with weight loss. The decline in protein consumption mixed with healthy meals is a simple way to cut excess weight and fat. Yet, there is an array of other benefits the vegan diet offers:

1 - Aids weight loss

Many people turn to the vegan diet to shed excess weight. Most studies state that vegans are lower in weight and BMI than non-vegans. These studies also suggest that the vegan diet is the best for weight loss than most other popular diets (40).

This is true for the calorie-restricted diet. Studies prove this. Even when a vegan eats until full, they lose more weight than those who controlled their calories. This is due to vegans choosing healthier lifestyle choices. Such as more exercise, less junk food, and healthier behavior.

Moreover, vegan meals tend to be higher in fiber.

Fibrous foods help you feel fuller for longer which helps with appetite control.

2 - Lowers the risk of cancer

The World Health Organisation (WHO) states that certain diets can lower the risk of cancer. Diets can prevent around one-third of all cancers (41).

The vegan diet includes many cancer reducing foods. Such as legumes, fruits, and vegetables. Vegans consume more of these foods than non-vegans. This is as they work well as substitutes for non-vegan foods (42).

Scientific studies have researched legumes. They concluded that they can reduce the risk of colorectal cancer by up to 18% (43). Moreover, fruits and vegetables can inhibit death from cancer by up to 15% (44).

Other studies suggest that soy products can reduce the risk of cancers. This includes prostate, breast, and colon. Soy products increase hormone receptors. This can help lower the chance of developing these cancers. Or, they can slow the progression, and decrease the severity (45).

It is still inconclusive of how much of each vegan food can lower the risk of developing such cancers.

3 - Reduces the risk of type 2 diabetes

The high fiber intake of the vegan diet reduces the need for sugary, and high carb foods. The reduction in sugary foods lowers the risk of insulin issues. High fiber foods can also blunt the effects sugar can have on insulin.

Studies suggest that vegan diets increase insulin sensitivity. This is beneficial for type 2 diabetic patients. This is as they suffer from poor insulin sensitivity. This study concludes that the vegan diet may be able to reduce the risk of type 2 diabetes by up to 78% (46).

4 - Improves heart health

The vegan diet seems to be able to regulate, and lower blood pressure. Which is beneficial for improved heart health.

A study on random individuals who adopted the vegan diet reduced their blood pressure by up to 78% (47). The same study found it may also be able to reduce the risk of heart disease by almost half.

These impressive results show how the vegan diet has a great effect on heart health.

Research also reveals that vegans have a lower LDL reading. LDL is bad cholesterol, and a lower LDL helps improve cholesterol. This study states that results are better with low sugar intake alongside the vegan diet (48).

5 - Reduces symptoms of arthritis

There have been new studies investigating the effects of the vegan diet on arthritis. Most reports show that the vegan diet can reduce the symptoms, and pain that arthritis can cause. This is due to vegan diets being rich in probiotics. Which are effective at reducing arthritis symptoms.

One study in particular studied 40 individuals that adopted a vegan diet for 6 weeks. All participants found an increase in energy. They also had improved the functioning of arthritic joints after consuming a vegan diet (49).

Arthritis patients report reduced swelling, pain, and improved mobility of the affected joints.

6 - Decreases the risk of poor kidney function

For those with current diabetes, the vegan diet may decrease the risk of poor kidney function.

One study found that diabetic vegan patients saw a decrease in the risk of poor kidney function. In particular, soy protein substitutes contributed to the efficacy of the vegan diet (50).

The vegan diet may not decrease the risk of poor kidney function better than non-vegan diets. Yet, it may still have some effect.

7 - Reduces the risk of Alzheimer's disease

The rate of Alzheimer's disease is increasing worldwide. Scientists are still researching the best methods for reducing the risk of this. Especially dietary changes.

These studies investigated the vegan diet to see the effect it has on the disease. Studies saw that plant-based products are better for neurological function (51). More than animal products. In particular, vegan diets are the most reliant on plant products. Hence, a vegan diet can help lower the risk of Alzheimer's disease.

The disease is often associated with a high intake of animal products and high-fat dairy. The vegan diet prohibits the consumption of animal products. Hence, justifying why the diet is beneficial for reducing the risk of this disease.

FAQ

I f you have any more concerns about the vegan diet. Then, here are answers to the top questions:

Do vegans lose weight faster?

Vegans are often thinner with a lower BMI than meat-eaters. This is usually down to the high fiber intake which helps curb cravings and control appetite. Also, plant-based substitutes can be healthier than animal product options. The vegan diet is among those with the quickest weight loss results. Research has concluded that the vegan diet is a more effective weight-loss tool. More so than meat-eating diets.

What is a good vegan breakfast?

There are many good vegan breakfast options. If you want it to be healthier, and a good energy source then pancakes, oats, and tofu are good options. You can make meals dairy-free with dairy substitutes. Any foods high in fiber will help increase energy and is sustainable.

Is peanut butter vegan?

Most peanut butter is vegan. It is often made with ground peanuts and salt. Yet, some are not vegan friendly as they use dairy butter. Always check the ingredients and labeling.

Can vegans eat cake?

Yes, vegans can eat cake. As long as they use non-dairy products.

Do vegans eat cheese?

Vegans can eat dairy-free cheeses. There are plenty of them on the market. From dairy-free mozzarella, and cheddar to vegan cream cheeses.

Can vegans eat bread?

Bread is often made with vegan-friendly products. Most consist of yeast, flour, water, and salt. But, there are some brands that add dairy, whey, or eggs which makes them non-vegan. Always read the labels to check for non-vegan ingredients.

Do vegans live longer?

According to studies, vegans have a 15% lower chance of dying without cause (52). The plant-based diet can increase longevity. This is due to the exclusion of animal chemicals, and toxins.

Vegans often choose healthier lifestyle choices, which may add to this.

Can vegans drink alcohol?

The majority of alcohol is vegan. All spirits are vegan. But, some wines and liquors can be non-vegan due to the addition of animal-based ingredients. Such as honey or isinglass. Or, some companies use a non-vegan friendly filtering process before bottling. Which involves animal products. Thus, it is not vegan friendly.

Do vegans eat potatoes?

All potatoes are vegan friendly. They are a ground vegetable. All vegetables are vegan friendly.

Do vegans poop more?

Vegans often consume more fiber than non-vegans. Fiber is a nutrient that can increase bowel movement. Thus, vegans may experience going to the toilet more often. It is not a bad thing. Fiber makes bowel movements more regular. This is a positive sign of a healthy digestive system.

Do vegans age quicker?

Protein is the key source to improve skin's elasticity. A lack of protein can cause poor elasticity. Thus, can excel in the aging process. Ensuring you eat enough plant-based protein will reduce the aging process. It can also improve your skin.

. . .

Veganism is growing in popularity quicker than ever. It is a worldwide diet that is often seen as a lifestyle. The elimination of all animal products is better for the environment and your body. It is a more sustainable, and ethical way of living. Hence, why many choose the diet for their body as much as the sustainability of the earth.

The vegan diet offers many health benefits. From improved heart health, weight loss, and reducing neurological conditions. A well-balanced nutrient-dense vegan diet is a very healthy way of eating. Plant-based foods are now, more than ever, easy to buy. There is a multitude of protein substitutes. Which allows a vegan to get their essential protein requirements.

With the right knowledge, and plan, it is simple to practice veganism.

Another diet more popular than ever is the keto diet. Very different from the vegan diet. Yet, offers more incredible health benefits. More on this to follow.

PART III

KETO DIET 101

"Non-violence leads to the highest ethics, which is the goal of all evolution. Until we stop harming all other living beings, we are still savages."

— Thomas A. Edison

1

WHAT IS THE KETO DIET?

T he keto diet is not a newfound diet. It has been
around since the 1920s and was then called the
ketogenic diet. Some still refer to it as the ketogenic diet today. "Keto" is a shortened version of the original name.

The ketogenic diet was first introduced as a treatment
for epilepsy. This was the original keto diet. Epileptic
patients found that high carbohydrate consumption wors-
ened their side effects. It also increased the risk of developing epilepsy. The patient has a 4:1 ratio of fat to protein
and carbs. 90% of the calories were from fat, 6% from
protein, and 4% from carbs.

Since it is profound for its many other health benefits.
The keto diet is often known for its weight loss and heart
health benefits. Yet, it also offers other benefits. This
includes reducing cholesterol, treating brain disorders, and
lowering blood sugar levels.

The keto diet is a very low carbohydrate and high-fat
diet. It limits carbohydrate intake, which allows room for

more fats, and proteins. This also encourages quick weight loss. Fat, and protein are great for providing energy. They are also the reason for the diet being very beneficial for your health.

2

HOW DOES THE KETO DIET WORK?

K eto suggests you should get about 80 percent of your daily calories from fat. Then, 20 percent from protein, and 10 percent from carbohydrates.

On the keto diet, fat is your friend. The substitution of fat allows the body to burn fat instead of glucose. This fat burning process is a metabolic state known as ketosis. Ketosis is beneficial for burning fat, and weight loss.

The keto diet promotes many health benefits such as:

- Weight loss
- Helping with diabetes - especially type 2 diabetic patients
- Reducing epileptic seizures
- Lowering the risk of neurological diseases - Alzheimer's, and Parkinson's disease
- Reducing the development of polycystic ovary syndrome (PCOS)
- Helping with brain injuries

- Lowering the risk of acne

The diet does not necessarily inhibit the conditions. More so it reduces symptoms and can help treat them. A keto diet is known to be best effective with heart health, and neurological diseases. More detail on these benefits, and studies is in the following chapters.

For best results, you must stick to the nutrient ratio, and consume keto-friendly foods. Without the right diet, there will be a lower chance of results. More on what to eat, and avoid for the keto diet is next.

3

WHAT TO EAT, AND AVOID ON THE KETO DIET?

T he elimination of carbohydrates with the increase in fat can help in many other ways. Eating the right foods will increase these health benefits.

The keto diet promotes eating lots of protein, low carb vegetables, and high-fat everything. The fat requirements are quite high. Fats you consume should always be healthy fats. These are best for the body and are those that promote health benefits.

The keto diet is 100% achievable whilst being vegan, which is what this section will cover. We will explain everything you need to know before trying the vegan keto diet.

Foods that are great for the keto diet include:

1- Unprocessed low carb meats

Replace your low-fat meats with high-fat meats. In the keto diet, it is important to reiterate that fats are your friend. Fats are good. High-quality meats offer many benefits and are those that are high in good fats. This includes grass-fed beef and venison. Pork is also a good option.

But remember, you do not need too much protein. Excess protein can convert into glucose, which you do not want to occur on the keto diet. Thus, you do not, and should not eat meat at every meal. Once a day is enough.

2 - Poultry

Other meats you can enjoy include poultry. This includes chicken and turkey. Any poultry is fine for the keto diet. Poultry contains less fat than red meats. It contains fewer calories as it is a leaner meat. Thus, if you are only eating meat once a day, and need to fit in lots of high-fat meat, red meat may be a better option. But, if you wish to eat meat twice a day, and not exceed the protein rule, poultry is a good option.

3 - Fish, and seafood

All fish and seafood are good to eat on the keto diet. Especially fatty fish like salmon. Salmon, among other fatty fish, contain lots of essential nutrients, and vitamins., and, they are very low in carbohydrates.

Fatty fish are high in omega-3's. Omega-3's are full of health benefits. Studies show that they can help reduce insulin levels and increase insulin sensitivity. This is very beneficial for diabetic patients, especially those who are overweight (53).

Salmon and omega-3's fatty fish also promote benefits for mental health (54). They can also reduce the risk of disease.

If you worry about toxins or mercury in large fish, there are plenty of smaller fish options. This includes herring and mackerel. Both great options for the keto diet.

4 - Eggs

Eggs are an easy way to get protein and healthy fats. One egg contains around 7 to 9 grams of protein and 5 grams of fat. They are also very low in carbohydrates. All which is perfect for the keto diet,

An egg is the most nutrient-dense food on the planet. Because of this, they are very filling. Studies show that eggs can help control appetite, and help you feel fuller for longer (55). You can enjoy them at every meal. They are a great addition to toast, salads, and bakes.

The great thing is, you eat them any way you want. Boiled, poached, fried, or scrambled. If you choose to cook them in anything other than water, there are a few healthy fats to suggest.

5 - Natural fats

Fats are a key part of the keto diet. There are many to choose from when it comes to cooking. This includes olive oil, coconut oil, avocado oil, and sesame oil. These are all high in natural fats which is good for the keto diet.

Natural fats are beneficial for heart health, anti-aging, and inflammation (56). A study shows how avocado oil can reduce the risk of heart conditions such as strokes, and diabetes (57).

As well as using them to cook, you can add oils to top your foods. Drizzling olive oil over vegetables or salads is a great way to increase your daily fat intake.

6 - High-fat sauces

As well as natural fats, high-fat sauces are fine on the keto diet. Seeing as most calories on the keto diet should come from fats, adding fats to the side of each meal is ideal. But, only healthy fats.

Avoid high sugar sauces, and substitute those for high-fat sauces. This includes bearnaise sauce, garlic sauce, lemon butter sauce, and no sugar mayonnaise. Sauces are great for low carbohydrate meals as fat helps you feel fuller for longer. Sauces also add flavor, and substance to food.

7 - Condiments, and spices

Talking of adding more flavor to your food. Condiments and spice are a great way to flavor your meals. Those that are okay on the keto diet are salt, pepper, and a few herbs. Those herbs include thyme, paprika, oregano, and cayenne.

The reason for only a few herbs fine for the keto diet is because of many herbs' external sugar. Extra sugar means carbohydrates. It is important to read into the sugar content before consuming such foods. This is as they some-times include hidden carbohydrates.

8 - Low carb vegetables

Herbs and vegetables can also contain hidden carbohy-drates. Many starchy vegetables like potatoes, corn, and squash are high in carbohydrates. Which, you should avoid.

Low carbohydrate vegetables are those that grow above ground. Or, are leafy green. This includes many vegeta-bles. Such as broccoli, cauliflower, kale, spinach, tomatoes, mushrooms, peppers, cabbage, and zucchini.

Many low carb vegetables, like mushrooms, and bell peppers, hold impressive anti-inflammatory properties.

This is ideal for reducing the risk of inflammation diseases. Such as gut issues, heart conditions, and chronic inflammation. Anti-inflammatory properties can also slow down aging, and improve brain function (58).

To make them even more keto diet appropriate, pour plenty of oil on them to add to the fat content. This will also add flavor.

9 - High-fat dairy

Let's make a point here that again, fat is your friend. High-fat dairy is often a food to avoid on diets. This is because people associate high-fat foods with weight gain. But, the right high-fat dairy options are very beneficial for weight loss. They also help you maintain a healthy keto diet.

Butter, high-fat dairy creams, and yogurts are ideal for the keto diet. They are also good for cooking. Both of which are also low in carbohydrates. Don't fear fat. Add butter, yogurts, and creams to your meals to increase daily fat intake.

Studies show that high-fat yogurts have great benefits for digestive health (59). It can repair, and maintain good gut health. It does this by fighting off bad bacterias.

More keto diet approved dairy is cheese. But, you have to be careful about which cheese you choose. Some cheeses are very high in carbohydrates. Crumbly dense cheeses contain more fat and fewer carbohydrates. The keto diet allows cheddar cheese, blue cheese, and feta cheese. Sometimes full fat cottage cheese is okay in small amounts. Again, cheese is a great addition to flavor and adds fat to many meals.

Yet, not all high-fat dairy is keto-approved. Such as milk. Avoid too much milk as milk can contain a lot of sugar. Sugar is carbohydrates, which is not okay on the keto diet.

10 - Seeds, and nuts

Seeds and nuts are great options as snacks for the keto diet. They are best to consume in moderation as they can make you exceed your daily carbohydrate limit. A handful a day of the following is fine.

Seeds accepted on the keto diet include pumpkin seeds, flaxseed, chia seeds, and hemp seeds.

For nuts, cashews are quite high in carbs. Thus, the best nut options include macadamia, pecan, almond, and brazil nuts.

Studies show that nuts and seeds are beneficial for insulin sensitivity (60). For example, one study shows that consuming pecans for one month improves insulin sensitivity (61).

Chia seeds are also great to consume daily. This is as they hold impressive anti-inflammatory properties. Studies suggest that chia seeds promote weight loss (62). They also offer anti-inflammation benefits. This helps for conditions such as heart attacks, and chronic inflammation. Remember to eat nuts, and seeds in moderation to prevent overloading on carbohydrates.

11 - Berries

Fruits are nature's candy. Most fruits are high in sugar, which can increase their carbohydrate content. Thus, not all fruits are okay for the keto diet.

Fruits that do work with the keto diet are red berries, as they contain the least sugar. Strawberries and raspberries are the lowest in sugar. As the sugar content is quite high for such a small food, you should eat them in moderation. Around half to a full cup of berries is acceptable each day.

12 - Avocados

Avocados are a fruit. They are very low in sugar, unlike most fruits. Plus, they are very high in healthy fats and low in carbohydrates. Making them perfect for the keto diet.

Avocados can be a great addition to any meal. They are ideal to eat around the clock. Avocados are full of essential vitamins, and nutrients such as folate, vitamin C, and K.

13 - Drinks

Many soft and alcoholic beverages are full of sugar. On the keto diet, glucose, and sugars are not okay.

Water is perfect. As we all know that water contains zero calories and sugars. You should consume around 2 to 3 liters of water per day.

Tea and coffee are good for the keto diet. As long as they do not contain milk or sugar. It is fine to add a small amount of milk to either but added sugar, and sweeteners are not allowed on the keto diet.

Bone broth is another liquid many like to consume on the keto diet. Not only is it hydrating, but bone broth is also filling, and full of essential nutrients, and fat.

For alcohol, you should avoid it almost completely. Yet, the occasional glass of wine is fine, if it is red. Red wine is best because the red berry content means it contains the least amount of sugar. This makes it lower in carbohydrates which are best for the keto diet.

. . .

With plenty of foods on the list, there is an extensive amount of flavor to enjoy. Ensure your meals are full of fat, and protein and low in carbs. Once you find your favorite foods from the list and create meals, it will be easier to sustain.

As well as foods to enjoy, there is also a list of foods to avoid on the keto diet.

4

FOODS TO AVOID

Most foods to avoid are self-explanatory and obvious. But, there are a few foods you need to avoid on the keto diet which may surprise.

- **Breaded meats, poultry, and fish:** crumbed meats and fish are high in carbohydrate
- **Cold cuts:** cold cuts of meats contain added sugar
- **Milky drinks:** coffees, hot chocolates, and teas
- **Low-fat yogurts:** fat is your friend on keto. Swap low-fat dairy products for high-fat as you need to consume as much fat as you can
- **Bread, and baked goods:** carbohydrates are a limited source of food on the keto diet. This category includes baked goods such as donuts, crackers, and rolls
- **Rice:** cooked rice contains starch which is carbohydrates

- **Pasta:** spaghetti and noodles are high in carbohydrates, which is not ideal for the keto diet
- **Starchy vegetables:** potatoes, sweet potatoes, peas, corn, pumpkin, squash. Swap these for above ground or leafy green vegetables to lower carbohydrate intake
- **Alcoholic beverages**: Beer, mixed drinks, and wines. They are all high in sugar
- **Sweetened beverages**: soda and juice are high in sugar. They are okay in small amounts
- **Candy**: sugar, ice cream, syrups, and chocolate. They are very high in sugar, Swap sweet treats for berries or no sugar/milk teas to please your cravings
- **Fruits**: citrus fruits, grapes, bananas, and pineapples. They are all high in sugar and net carbohydrates. Substitute these with a small number of berries
- **High carb sauces**: barbeque sauce, sugary salad dressings, ketchup, honey mustard, and dipping sauces. They are all very high in carbohydrates. Substitute these for buttery low carb sauces
- **Unhealthy fats**: vegetable oils, corn oil, margarine all contain unhealthy fats. Swap these for olive oil, avocado oil or coconut oil to consume healthier, and more natural fats
- **Processed foods**: ready-made meals, fast food, and packaged food
- **Diet foods**: any that contain added preservatives or sweeteners

Use these lists as a guide for shopping. Consuming the right foods will help you stay on track, and achieve the best results the keto diet offers.

5

FAQ

T o become a pro on the keto diet, you may be wondering a few more things. To add to your knowledge, here are some answers to the top questions:

What is a good breakfast for fasting on the keto diet?

A typical keto breakfast should include high-fat, plant protein, and no carbs. Any type of tofu is ideal for a keto diet. For example, tofu scramble omelets are a good option. These can be cooked with low carb vegetables. Such as mushrooms, tomatoes, kale, peppers, and spinach. Or, a cooked breakfast that includes tofu, avocado, tomatoes, and vegetables is a good option.

Low carb options are the best to break a fast as it will inhibit a spike in blood sugar levels.

Is peanut butter keto?

Peanut butter is acceptable on keto. But, only if it is natural peanut butter. As those are quite low in carbs. All peanut butter are high-fat due to the peanuts inside. Yet, some can contain added sugars. Thus, always opt for natural peanut butter to avoid excess carbs.

Can you eat bananas on keto?

Bananas are very high in carbs for such a small piece of food. One medium banana contains around 24 grams of carbs. Thus, they are not good for the keto diet. For a fruit serving, red berries are a better option. They contain around 5 to 7 grams of carbs per half or full cup.

Can you drink alcohol on keto?

You can drink one glass of red wine, and stay in ketosis. Yet, if you do this often it can slow down progress, and results. Beers and mixed sugary drinks are high in carbs. They are not good for the keto diet.

Can you drink Coke Zero on keto?

Coke Zero does not contain carbs or sugars. Thus, it should not affect ketosis. But, if you drink it often, it can slow down progress, and also has a knock-on effect on your health.

Can I have cheat days on keto?

A cheat day is not accepted on a keto diet. Cheat days will spike your blood sugar, and decrease your progress. If you feel the need to give in to your cravings, opt for vegan keto accepted foods.

Can I snack on keto?

There are many snacks that are keto accepted. This includes high-fat low carb snacks. Such as kale chips, olives, avocados, nuts, seeds, low carb vegetables, eggs, and yogurts. Avoid sugary snacks such as candy, and high carb fruits.

Can you stay on keto forever?

Keto dieting is good for the long term, but not forever. This is due to the high-fat content of the diet. But, healthy fats do offer many health benefits. Eating them a lot forever may have a knock-on effect. There is not enough evidence to say that staying on keto forever is good or bad. It may be better to dip in, and out of the keto diet if you want to sustain it forever.

What color is your pee in ketosis?

A change of color in your pee can sometimes occur on the keto diet. This is because the ketosis process may make you dehydrated, which can cause your pee to turn yellow. Stay hydrated to prevent this.

So long as you stick to the daily nutritional intakes, you can sustain the keto diet. This should not exceed more than 70% of your calories from fat, 20% from protein, and 10% from carbohydrates. Tracking your carbohydrate intake is very helpful. It helps you to not exceed 45 grams per day limit.

Substitute carbohydrates for high-fat foods. Healthy natural fats are a great addition to any meal and are an ideal way to increase your daily fat intake.

With this food list and top tips, it is easier than ever to start and maintain a keto diet. One that offers many health benefits. Plus, it is a great one to encourage you to sustain the diet as a lifestyle to continue reaping the benefits.

Vegan and keto are now popular diets together. The vegan keto diet is a new diet many people are using to maximize health benefits. The keto diet does promote the consumption of animal products. Which the vegan diet does not. But, it is simple to substitute the protein, and fat requirements. To learn more about it, its benefits, and how to try it yourself, read on for the ultimate guide.

PART IV

VEGAN KETO DIET 101

"I've found that a person does not need protein from meat to be a successful athlete. In fact, my best year of track competition was the first year I ate a vegan diet."

— Carl Lewis

1

WHAT IS VEGAN KETO DIET?

Many dieting techniques associate restricting carbohydrates, and sugars for weight loss. Limiting those foods is very beneficial for weight loss. But, there are many more health benefits that are on offer from cutting out certain foods.

Combining two diets can be successful. It is also very popular. It allows a person to achieve more benefits, such as helping with medical issues. A popular combination diet is the vegan keto diet. All of which this guide is for.

The vegan keto diet follows a low carbohydrate and plant-based plan.

The vegan diet is often high in carbohydrates, which keto is not. This can sometimes make it difficult for a vegan to follow a keto diet. Yet, a meal plan that restricts all the necessary foods makes it more simple than you think. Plus, it offers many great health benefits.

2

HISTORY OF THE VEGAN KETO DIET

The vegan keto diet is a new and modernized diet which became popular in the past decade. The history of the two diets combined does not date back far. Yet, the two diets have existed by themselves for much longer.

This is due to the uncertainty of the safety, and health benefits. Also, both are new diets for the health industry. Neither had much research behind them to verify their benefits. Yet today, there is much more scientific knowledge of how to sustain the diets in a healthy way.

The keto diet was popular during the 1920s when used as a treatment for epilepsy. Later, the keto diet was outshone by other diets from the Atkins diet to fasting.

In the late 1960s through to the 1970s, the keto diet was reborn due to research on the process of ketones. Scientists found that low carbohydrate meals were easy to replace. This is with healthy fats and high protein. The nutrients found in these foods are a more sustainable energy source. Then, the discovery of the keto diets health benefits began.

The vegan diet was a more commercialized diet. This is due to it being existent but not defined for a long time. Then, in the 1940's it was known as the vegan diet. Sometimes mistaken for the vegetarian diet. These diets are very different as vegans cut consumption of all animal products. This includes eggs, dairy products, and honey. Before veganism, people knew it as the non-dairy vegetarian diet. Now, it is the vegan diet.

3

HOW TO COMBINE VEGAN + KETO?

To begin the vegan keto diet, it is important to understand how it works. It is as important to also understand how to combine the diets for them to work to their full effect.

The rules for the vegan diet are simple. It is important to cut the consumption of animal products. Eating animal products is not acceptable. This includes more than meat and fish. Eggs, dairy, and any other product from an animal are not for consumption. Even honey from a bee is not acceptable on a vegan diet. Although this sounds like a lot to cut, this book will be your guide. Substituting animal products with plant-based products is very simple. We will help you understand what to avoid, and substitute to achieve a 100% vegan keto diet.

For the keto diet part of this combination diet, you need to limit your carbohydrate intake. Do not consider only grains, wheat, and rye products to be carbohydrates. For example, carbohydrates include more than bread, pasta, cereals, and potatoes. Vegetables and fruits can have a high carbohydrate content due to the sugars present. It is important to be aware of the number of carbs you are consuming each day and limit it. More on the limits and restrictions are to follow.

Below are a few things that need to ensure you are following the correct vegan keto diet dietary requirements:

- Consume at least 70% of your calories from plant-based fats
- Remove meat, fish, dairy, eggs, and all animal products from your diet
- Limit carbohydrate intake to 45 grams a day or less
- Eat low carbohydrate vegetables over high carb
- Consume 25% of your calories from plant-based proteins
- Ensure you are getting the nutrients you are missing out on through supplements. This includes vitamin D's, and B's, irons, zinc, and taurine

More information on what foods to eat, and what foods to avoid is to follow. This will help you with limiting your intake of certain food groups., and, will also help you find protein plant-based substitutes.

Keto and vegan diets have very strict limitations. These are important to stick by to achieve the benefits and results.

4
___

THE IMPORTANCE OF SUPPLEMENTS, AND DIET QUALITY

The diets alone can cause some nutrient deficiencies. Vegan and keto diets restrict different foods. Yet, both are deficient in some essential nutrients, and vitamins. Thus, when put together this can cause further nutrient deprivation.

Do not starve your body, and deprive it of nutritional foods. Creating a meal plan is the best way to dictate what you will eat, and when. Meal planning will help you see what nutrients you are missing out on. Thus, it will help you to consume all the daily nutrients your body needs.

As this is a restrictive diet there are many foods that can replace cravings and nutrients. When starting the vegan keto diet, you should try lots of different foods to find out what works for you. Experimenting with plant-based protein supplements is a key step.

For the keto diet, eating enough protein is essential. The daily protein intake replaces the energy that before-hand would come from carbohydrates.

But, vegans often lack protein in their diets due to the elimination of animal products. This may seem an issue for combining the two diets. As one requires food the other has to avoid. But, it is easy to source protein from plants. There are many high protein vegan alternatives such as soy products, and nuts.

It is important to eat a quality diet with high-quality foods on the vegan keto diet. Avoiding a high-quality diet may impact your health. Lack of nutrients can cause deficiencies that impact more than your energy levels.

For example, lacking in iron is an issue for vegans. This is because most iron-rich foods are meat, and fish, which vegans do not eat. Thus, replacing iron in the diet is essential. Iron deficiency can cause your tissues, and muscles to deplete. They do not get enough oxygen without iron. This means they are not able to work well. This leads to a condition called anemia. To avoid this, supplements, and high-quality food substitutes are key.

If you want to stick to the vegan keto diet long term, it is best to ease into it. The food requirements are restrictive which can take some time to get used to. It may also take some people time to find the right substitutes, especially for the vegan part of the diet. Meat-eaters in particular may take longer.

Easing into it will allow your body to adjust to the new food routine and nutritional daily intakes. Lacking several essential nutrients at once may make your body go into shock. It may cause extreme fatigue or daily nausea. Easing into it can prevent this. Then, over time your body will understand what nutrients it is lacking. This is then where you should replace those nutrients with supplements.

5

10 SUPPLEMENTS YOU NEED ON A VEGAN DIET

Although a vegan diet is highly nutritious, it sometimes lacks certain essential vitamins. To combat nutrient and vitamin deficiencies, vegans can benefit from taking certain supplements that they may lack. The top 10 supplements the vegan diet can benefit from include:

1- Vitamin B12

Vitamin B12 is one of the crucial vitamins the vegan diet misses out on. This particular B vitamin is primarily found in animal products. As the vegan diet eliminates all animal produce, it eliminates the easy access to vitamin B12.

Vitamin B12 is a vitamin that helps manage and maintain many essential bodily functions. It can improve and increase healthy red blood cells, support the nervous system, increase fertility and metabolise proteins. Without this vitamin, these bodily functions can deteriorate and cause health issues.

Thus, it is important to ensure you have enough vitamin B12 in your diet. Especially for those that are vegan and can lack in this vitamin.

Studies show that vegans have dramatically lower vitamin B12 in their blood than consumers of animal produce. The study suggests taking a vitamin B12 supplement can easily increase levels.

Aside from supplements, there are other ways vegans can add vitamin B12 into their diet. Studies reveal that consumption of the following foods can improve vitamin B12 levels:

- Nori seaweed
- Nutritional yeast
- Mushrooms
- Soy products - tofu, beans and milk
- Breakfast cereals
- Spirulina
- Chlorella

The only way for vegans to reach the recommended daily intake of vitamin B12 of 2.4 mcg is to take supplements and add these foods into their daily diet.

2 - Vitamin D

Vitamin D is a fairly scarce source when it comes to food options. Hence, vegans can struggle to meet the daily vitamin D intake requirements.

It is an essential vitamin that typically promotes easy

absorption of calcium and phosphorus. Studies reveal that vitamin D can inhibit many health conditions from cancers to autoimmune diseases. It is a vitamin that expresses health amongst numerous parts of the body. Thus, without it the body can suffer and develop health issues.

Other vital functions of vitamin D include:

- Improving mood
- Helping with memory
- Maintaining healthy immune functioning
- Speeds up muscle recovery

Vitamin D typically comes from foods such as oily fish, eggs, red meats and fat spreads. All of which are prohibited on the vegan diet.

Other ways to increase vitamin D is with sun exposure. But, this is often heavily not recommended due to skin damage and negative effects of regular UV exposure.

Thus, taking a vitamin D supplement can greatly benefit vegans. Vitamin D is also promoted as a fortified vitamin in many plant based milks.

To check your vitamin D level, you can get a reading from a doctor. Healthy levels measure at 30 mg/dL or more. If your reading is below that, vegan or not, it is important and essential to take supplements to improve the reading. Not only will it benefit your mood, memory and muscle repair but healthy levels of vitamin D can inhibit the development of health conditions.

3 - Iron

Anemia is a common problem for vegan diets. This is simply an iron deficiency. Iron is a key vitamin for healthy functioning of red blood cells, which helps carry oxygen through the blood. Studies conclude that iron is also essential for energy absorption and metabolism.

Iron rich foods are categorised into two groups. One being heme, which comes from animal produce such as meat. Heme iron is easier to digest and contains a high concentration of iron. The second group is non heme which is derived from plants.

Plant based/non heme sources that are rich in iron include:

- Nuts - pistachios, brazil, almonds and cashews
- Legumes - beans, pea and lentils
- Whole grains - oatmeal, barley, rice, buckwheat and bulgar
- Dark leafy vegetables - spinach, kale, swiss chard and collard greens
- Dried fruits - peaches, prunes, currants, raisins and pears
- Seeds - pumpkin, flaxseed, sesame and hemp

Whilst these foods can maintain adequate levels of iron for vegans, studies show that some may still develop a deficiency. Taking an iron supplement can combat and prevent a deficiency to help maintain healthy functioning of cells.

Consuming too much iron can cause other medical issues. For an iron level reading, consult your doctor. From the reading, they will suggest whether or not an iron supplement is necessary.

4 - Omega-3 fatty acids

Omega-3's are essential fatty acids that derive from a variety of foods. There are two types of omega-3's. The first are essential omega-3 fatty acids which you can only get from your diet. These foods are known as ALA's and can be easily consumed by vegans as they are from plant based food sources such as seeds and soybeans.

However, the second type of omega-3 are long chain omega-3 fatty acids, which vegans can easily lack. There are two forms of long chain fatty acids, EPA and DHA. Although these are not essential, they are found to be crucial for brain and cardiovascular health. Long chain omega-3's can reduce the risk of many diseases from cancers and inflammation to mental disorders. EPA and DHA are most often derived from fatty fish and their oils. Hence, they are not vegan friendly.

Long chain omega-3's can be maintained through adequate amounts of ALA. But not for all vegans. Research has discovered that vegans typically have 50% less long chain fatty acids in their blood than non-vegans. Thus, taking long chain omega-3 fatty acid supplements can improve this quantity and promote good health and disease prevention.

5 - Iodine

Iodine is a vitamin which is often hard to maintain if your diet eliminates animal produce. This is due to foods high in iodine being grown on farms or in the ocean. These include fish, dairy products and salts.

As vegans lack these foods, they can easily become iodine deficient. Iodine is crucial for thyroid metabolism and can prevent hyperthyroidism. This is an issue that can cause issues for pregnant women and from that, can stunt infants growth. In rare cases, it can cause infant disability. Studies found that symptoms of hyperthyroidism are commonly fatigue, dry skin, weight gain and depression.

To prevent becoming iodine deficient, it is recommended for vegans to take supplements daily. Iodine can be consumed from seaweed in high quantities. Or, fortified foods can be iodized, but are more often than not very unhealthy. So, if you do not wish to consume seaweed or fortified foods daily, supplements are the best option.

6 - Calcium

The calcium vitamin plays an important role in bone health. It can also improve the health of the muscles, teeth, heart and nerves. Without it, these body parts can suffer and be at risk of disease.

Calcium rich foods are typically meat and dairy. For vegans, plant based options can provide a decent amount of calcium. But, not as adequate as animal products. Plant based sources of calcium include:

- Kale
- Mustard greens
- Bok choy
- Chickpeas
- Broccoli
- Calcium set tofu

- Fortified milks

The recommended daily intake of calcium is 1,000mg. Research suggests that individuals who consume less than 500mg of calcium daily can have a high risk of bone fracture. If a vegan finds they are lacking in calcium, eating plant based sources and taking supplements is advised.

7 - Zinc

Zinc plays an important role in the body. It is a mineral which acts as a stimulant for over 100 enzymes in the body. It can improve immune function, metabolism and gene regulation. As well as that, zinc can combat chronic disease and inflammation.

With there being very few plant food sources being rich in zinc, it is highly recommended to take daily supplements.

Plant based zinc food sources include whole grains, tofu, legumes, seeds and nuts. These foods can increase zinc intake but may not help a vegan reach the daily average intake. The average intake of zinc is 8 to 11 mg. Studies reveal that non-omnivores have a considerably lower zinc reading than omnivores. So, a daily supplement to meet the daily requirement is advised.

8 - Vitamin K2

There are two types of vitamin K that the body needs for healthy functioning. Vitamin K1 is found in dark leafy green, which is appropriate for the plant based diet. Vitamin K2 can be found in some plant based sources such as fermented soy and vegetables dishes. But, vitamin K2 is typically found in dairy products and egg yolks, which is prohibited from the vegan diet.

Both forms of vitamin K are essential for managing and digesting calcium. Those that lack in this crucial vitamin may have issues with bone density.

With there being very few vitamin K2 enriched plant based foods, supplements are an ideal method of increasing daily intake.

9 - Selenium

Selenium is a mineral that helps protect the body from neurodegenerative disorders and cardiovascular diseases. It is very rarely found in plant foods due to soil depletion. Selenium rich foods include red meats, poultry, fish and eggs. Therefore, it can be difficult for the vegan diet to acquire selenium.

The highest selenium plant based food is brazil nuts. Thus, unless you wish to consume brazil nuts with most meals, supplements are an easy way to maintain healthy levels of selenium.

10 - Magnesium

The magnesium mineral can be easily lacked in the vegan diet. Again, due to soil depletion. It is essential to have good levels of magnesium as it helps with iodine absorption, muscle and nerve regulation. If you plan to take iodine supplements it would be beneficial to take magnesium to.

Foods rich in magnesium include non-vegan friendly options such as dairy foods and meat.

But, there are a few plant based options that are vegan

friendly such as nuts, brown rice, leafy greens and whole grain.

If you wish to maintain healthy magnesium levels, consuming these foods daily alongside supplements will be highly beneficial.

6

BENEFITS OF THE VEGAN KETO DIET

The vegan keto diet is one of the most challenging diets as it is quite restrictive. But, is it manageable with the right food plan, and sustainable food choices. It also offers many health benefits.

The diets as a combination are quite new. So, there is not yet enough evidence for the health benefits. Yet, there was a 6-month study for random participants who consumed the vegan keto diet. This found that all had significant weight loss (63). They also had a reduction in cholesterol and triglycerides. All are beneficial for many health conditions such as diabetes. These findings are also beneficial for heart disease. This is as high cholesterol levels are the key cause of heart disease.

Moreover, there is plenty of research for the diets on their own. Which further explores more benefits they can deliver.

Helps with weight loss

If weight loss is your main goal for choosing the vegan keto diet, much research verifies that. Both diets promote weight loss due to the restriction of food groups.

In particular, keto diets are profound for its weight loss benefits. This is due to its reduction in carbohydrates. Without the heavy consumption of carbohydrates, the body goes into a state of ketosis. This is where the body burns fat for fuel instead of carbohydrates. As the body will not be consuming many carbohydrates, there will be little carbs to use for energy. Thus, your body will look to use the second reserve, which is fat. Burning fat is essential for weight loss.

There are many studies on vegan diets for their weight loss successes. Studies found that vegans have lower body fat mass, and BMI than non-vegans (64). This is further proven by a study that found that vegans have an easier ability to lose weight (65). They also find it easier to sustain a healthy weight due to the increase in glycemic control. Which, is due to the food choices in the diet. The blood sugar levels down helping a person lose weight, and maintain it.

Both diets promote weight loss, and evidence proves they can both benefit in that area of dieting. Thus, this diet is a good option for those who wish to lose weight. It is important to be aware that there are other, and more health-promoting benefits.

Lowers the risk of high blood pressure

A study found that 96%of vegans have a 75% lower risk of getting high blood pressure (66). This is due to the elimination of animal products in the diet. Meats can be high in saturated fats, which are a key cause of high blood pressure, and reducing heart health.

The study found that veganism in men reduces the risk of high blood pressure more than women (67). Yet, there is not enough evidence to conclude why. But, both genders saw a reduction in the risk.

Studies on the keto diet for diabetic patients suggest that it can lower the risk of high blood pressure (68).

Reduces the risk or severity of type 2 diabetes

Many studies have found that vegans have a much lower risk of developing type 2 diabetes. This is due to the studies concluding in patients having lower blood sugar levels. One study found that vegan diets lower the risk of developing type 2 diabetes decreases by up to 78% (69).

A research study investigated the reason for vegans have a much lower risk of type 2 diabetes. The research found that it may be due to high fiber intake. Vegans eat a plant-based diet which involves a lot of high fiber foods such as vegetables, and fruits. Fiber works to cut blood sugar levels by reducing their response.

Furthermore, the keto diet has shown positive results for its insulin balancing benefits. One study found that diet can improve insulin sensitivity by up to 75%. This research found that 35% of type 2 diabetic patients could stop using medication. This is only whilst being on the keto diet, due to its insulin benefits (70).

Also, both diets promote weight loss. This is beneficial for those who need to lower blood sugar levels. As it can reduce the severity or risk of diabetes.

Lessens the risk/symptoms of cancer

Scientists study these diets on their own to discover the effects they have on cancer. Both are different in how they manage to help with cancer, but both conclude to be beneficial for cancer.

One study found that the food restrictions in the keto diet were effective as a therapy for brain cancer (71). The effects of the keto diet are more than 65% alike to medical therapies. It has since been an alternative or treatment method for brain cancer patients. Many of the patients follow a keto diet to reap these benefits.

An observational study found that veganism can reduce the risk of developing cancer by up to 15% (72). This is due to the benefits of blood sugar levels, and heart health. Thus, suggesting that a vegan diet can benefit cancers that are a result of bad heart health.

Slows the development of Alzheimer's Disease

The keto diet has a history of research for its effect on neurological conditions. Studies found that ketogenic dieting can have positive neuroprotective effects. The study found that the diet can help slow down the development, and severity of Alzheimer's disease (73). A low carb diet can boost the brain's functions and cognitive ability. This can influence the progression of a disease like Alzheimer's to slow down.

The vegan diet has benefits for Alzheimer's disease. This is as it can reduce the risk of developing the condition. Evidence suggests that animal products can influence neurological conditions like Alzheimer's (74). Thus, a nonanimal product diet can have positive effects. As it can limit the risk for such neurological conditions.

The foods consumed in a vegan keto diet are beneficial for brain health, and development. Hence why it is beneficial for a neurological condition like Alzheimer's disease.

There are other benefits of both diets which do not coincide with each other. But, by partaking in both diets, you can reap the separate benefits from both diets.

The keto diet can also help with other health conditions. This includes neurological conditions. Such as epilepsy, and Parkinson's disease. Other conditions include polycystic ovary syndrome (PCOS), and brain injuries. The diet may not inhibit the conditions, more so it reduces symptoms, and can help treat them. A keto diet is best effective with heart health, and neurological diseases. This is because there is more conclusive evidence that shows results.

For the vegan diet, other health benefits include arthritis and kidney functioning. The benefits here are not to inhibit or treat the conditions. Instead, the diet can help slow the progress and severity of the symptoms.

Some of the latter health benefits mentioned for both diets are not yet said to be 100% effective. But, there is evidence to suggest that the diets do have some effect on treating or reducing symptoms. By consuming the vegan keto diet, a person can reap the health benefits mentioned above.

7

RISKS OF THE VEGAN KETO DIET

A vegan keto is a very restrictive diet which means it may not work for everyone. Those who wish to try it, and see if it suits them may experience some side effects and risks.

Although the diet is plant-based, that does not mean it is the healthiest diet out there.

All diets have their drawbacks, and here are those for this diet.

The lack of animal products means that it lacks in a few essential vitamins, and nutrients. Our bodies need these nutrients to function to their full potential.

Studies show that nonanimal eaters can be deficient in many essential vitamins (75). This includes vitamin B12, iron, calcium, and zinc. To get these vitamins, it is advised to take supplements alongside the diet. This is to ensure you are getting all of the vitamins your body needs.

It is as important to eat healthy balanced meals. This should include enough protein, healthy fats, and carbo-hydrates.

The vegan keto diet may be difficult for those with

bowel issues. This is because it may be hard for those to digest certains foods. This may be even more so than a normal person. As plant-based proteins are harder to digest than animal proteins. Research states that plant-based proteins do not undergo sulfur muscle protein synthesis. Which makes it harder for the body to break down the protein. It can cause excess gas, bloating, or trouble going to the toilet.

Studies suggest that people may experience the keto flu when starting the diet. This involves the following side effects:

- Weakness
- Headaches
- Diarrhea
- Irritability
- Constipation
- Nausea
- Fatigue
- Poor concentration
- Muscle cramps
- Dizziness
- Trouble sleeping

You should drink plenty of water when easing into the diet. Also, rest, eat foods rich in fiber, take plenty of supplements your body may be lacking, and do not over-exercise.

This diet may not work for everyone, and that is normal. There are a few people who should not partake in this diet. This includes those with type 1 diabetes or eating disorders. Plus, pregnant or breastfeeding women. This is because the diet can be detrimental to their health. If you are unsure if the vegan keto diet will affect you, it is best to consult a doctor.

The vegan keto diet does come with many positives. It offers many health benefits., and, can help people live a healthier and more sustainable lifestyle. The Academy of Nutrition and Dietetics report that high-quality vegan diets are healthful (76).

8

THE ULTIMATE SHOPPING LIST GUIDE

With any diet, there are foods that you should consume, and foods advised to avoid.

The vegan keto diet advises the consumption of high-quality protein and fats. This should substitute carbohydrates. The keto diet should consist of low carbs meals. Although it may seem that combining the two food restrictive diets will lack a lot of exciting foods. That perception is wrong. There is an extensive list of foods that you can choose from.

First, it is important to consider protein. A vegan diet can often lack in protein if a person does not find protein-packed substitutes. Protein from animals is "complete" protein. This provides all essential amino acids a body needs to grow, and function well. Plant-based proteins are "incomplete" as they lack amino acids. But, over the years there have been plenty of new vegan protein options.

Then, you need to take into consideration the recommended carbohydrate intake. This is between 15, and 40 grams per day. It is important to be aware that carbohydrates are not high in grains, wheat, and starchy products. Many vegetables can be high in carbohydrates too.

Then, for both diets, you should eat as many healthy fats as possible over unhealthy fats. In the vegan keto diet, you should intake around 25% of your calories from protein. 70% or more from healthy fats, and the rest carbohydrates. With that in mind, here is a list of foods to eat:

- Plant-based high protein alternatives: tempeh, tofu, seitan
- Low carb vegetables: leafy greens, broccoli, cauliflower, zucchini, peppers, mushrooms, cucumber
- High-fat dairy alternatives: unsweetened coconut-based dairy (milk, and creams), vegan cheeses, vegan butter
- Nuts, seeds, and nut butter: pistachios, almonds, sunflower seeds, pumpkin seeds
- Fruits: raspberries, blackberries, avocados, and other low glycemic impact berries in small quantities
- Fermented foods: natto, sauerkraut, kim chi
- Sea vegetables: dulse, bladderwrack, kelp
- Condiments, and sweeteners: salt, and pepper. Spices, lemon juice, fresh herbs, stevia, erythritol, nutritional yeast
- Healthy fat oils: coconut oil, olive oil, MCT oil, avocado oil, macadamia oil, sesame oil
- Drinks: coffee, tea, water, healthy juices with the recommended fruit/low-carb vegetables

Eating plenty of these foods will help you get all the nutrition your body needs on a daily basis. You can consume them at every meal. You need to be aware of the amount you should eat to abide by the 25% protein, and 70% healthy fats recommendation. It is important to ensure your body gets enough protein. Thus, replacing animal products with soy products is a great, and plentiful alternative.

To ensure you are eating right for the diet, it is important to avoid certain foods. Below is a list of foods to not buy or consume during this diet.

- Grains: high carb wheat, rice, cereals, oats, quinoa, pasta
- Legumes: high carb lentils, beans, and chickpeas
- Starchy vegetables: carrots, corn, sweet potatoes, parsnips, peas, beetroot, squash
- Fruits: cherries, oranges, pears, grapefruit, dried apricot, strawberries, plums
- Dairy: milk, butter, yogurt
- Eggs: egg whites, and egg yolks
- Seafood: all seafood - fish, shrimp, clams, mussels
- Meat: all meat, and poultry - beef, turkey, chicken, pork
- Animal-based ingredients: honey, agave, whey protein, egg white protein
- Sugary foods: maple syrup, agave syrup, soda, juice, sauces, sports drinks
- Processed, and packaged foods
- Gelatin, and collagen products
- Alcohol

Writing up a shopping list, and meal planning before shopping can help you stay on track. Creating a plan is an easy way to understand what you should eat, and avoid. It should make the diet feel easier. Having the right foods in your fridge will encourage you to eat better. In time, this may influence you to sustain these eating habits long term.

With the right knowledge, and foods, the vegan keto diet is definitely a diet that can be a lifestyle.

Some people may have more concerns or questions. So, below are answers to the top asked questions on the vegan keto diet:

9

FAQ

Do you lose weight being vegan?

Most studies conclude that vegans lose more weight than non-vegans or vegetarians. But, only if they stick to the daily nutritional guidelines, and exercise often. It is also said that vegans have healthier BMI's, and less body fat than non-vegans (77).

Do you lose more weight on a keto or vegan diet?

There is no definite answer to which diet will achieve the most weight loss. It depends on the person and their current or previous diet.

Weight loss will occur if a person eats a lot of carbohydrates in their current diet. This is because the switch to a keto diet limits carb intake, which can affect weight.

The same happens for meat-eaters who eat a lot of saturated fatty meat, and dairy products. Such as bacon, steak, and cheese. Once a person removes these high in fat products, a person will lose body fat. Thus, they will lose weight.

A person's exercise routine and current diet will encourage how much weight a person can lose.

Can vegans eat pasta?

Most pasta is not manufactured from animal products. Thus, it is okay for vegans. Yet, some pasta use eggs. Thus, always check the ingredients list before consuming as eggs are not vegan.

Do vegans age quicker?

Any diet that lacks protein and healthy fats can cause an increase in aging. Thus, it is important to protein-packed plant-based foods to get enough protein. Protein in foods helps the skin's collagen and elasticity. Thus when consumption is less, it will cause aging.

Lacking in essential vitamins such as zinc, and omega-3's can also cause aging. Supplements help vegans get all the essential vitamins they miss out on. This will reverse the deficiency and aging process.

How much weight can you lose on the vegan keto diet?

How much weight a person can lose from being on the vegan keto diet depends on the change from the previous diet. If a person eliminates lots of foods in a short space of time, weight loss may be more significant.

Exercising often, and eating enough protein will help maintain healthy body weight. It will also ensure the body does not become too low on energy.

Is coffee vegan?

Coffee beans are from a plant. Thus, coffee is vegan. Consume black or with non-dairy milk such as coconut, almond, or soya to ensure it is 100% vegan.

Why am I gaining weight on a vegan diet?

Sometimes vegans lack in protein and substitute that with carbohydrates, and fats. This is a huge factor for weight gain. Be careful what you substitute your past foods for.

Combining the two diets will limit your carb and unhealthy fat intake. This should not encourage weight gain or poor food substitution.

What is the lowest carb fruit?

Berries are the most popular choice when it comes to low carb fruits. Strawberries have the lowest carb content. Berries, in small quantities, are often encouraged for the vegan keto diet. Carbs in fruit come from the high sugar content. It is important to understand that fruits and vegetables can have a high carb content. This is due to them being high in sugar.

Most diets cause some complications for certain individuals. So, it is important to address any complications for the vegan keto diet.

Complications of the Vegan Keto Diet (Gender, Age, and Medical)

Whilst there is very little risk for healthy individuals for the vegan keto diet. There are some complications to be aware of. The diet is safe for all genders, and ages, above 18 years old. Yet, there are more complications for women than for men.

The vegan keto diet does not offer better results for men than women. But, more risks can be a problem for women. This is due to the hormonal changes that can happen during the diet.

For example, nutrient deprivation can be damaging for a pregnant or breastfeeding woman. To grow a healthy baby, a woman must consume all essential nutrients. A baby needs all essential nutrients to function well during, and after birth. A lack of certain vitamins can impair a newborn baby's development.

For the same reason, a child should not partake in this diet. Nor should they partake in any restrictive diet. It can be damaging to elderly adults' health as much as a child. Not having proper knowledge or a high-quality diet can cause damage. Thus, children and the elderly should avoid the vegan keto diet.

Studies show it may not be beneficial for type 1 diabetic patients (78). This is due to the frequent changes in insulin levels. Type 1 diabetic patients find it more difficult to control and balance insulin than type 2. More so, type 1 diabetic patients do not have a cure for their diabetes. But, this diet can benefit type 2 diabetes as they can reverse the condition.

The combination of the diet may not offer any benefits for athletes. This is due to athletes having to prevent nutrient deficiencies to stay in the best shape. Lack of certain vitamins and food groups can decline their performance.

Anyone with previous or current eating disorders should also avoid the diet. Again, lack of nutrients and food restrictions can impact health and weight. Anyone that does not eat a high-quality diet already should not partake in a restrictive diet.

There is not yet any evidence to suggest that the diet can benefit one age or gender more than another. Thus, there are no specifics for men, women, and age groups to address.

Is Vegan Keto Possible?

The restrictiveness of this diet may have you questioning if this diet is possible. The conclusive answer is, definitely. The vegan keto diet is possible for anyone that has the right knowledge. It will work for anyone with no under-lying health issues.

Already there are many studies to suggest the vegan keto diet offers lots of benefits. It can help with weight loss and fat burning. It is even safe to be on this diet whilst fasting. Thus, suggesting it is a great diet to choose if you want to have a sustainable healthy lifestyle. The plant protein and fat substitutes are a great way of taking care of the world, and your body.

Having the right knowledge, and guidance is the key to success. Then, the main thing to reiterate is high-quality meals. Ensuring your body gets the essential makes the diet possible, and safe. The person partaking in the diet handles prohibiting any health deficiencies or dangers.

PART V

HOW TO COMBINE VEGAN KETO & INTERMITTENT FASTING

"By eating meat we share the responsibility of climate change, the destruction of our forests, and the poisoning of our air and water. The simple act of becoming a vegetarian will make a difference in the health of our planet."

— Thích Nhất Hạnh

1

WHY COMBINE VEGAN KETO WITH INTERMITTENT FASTING?

Vegan, keto, and fasting diets are all very popular. They all benefit from weight loss and other health conditions. Although all are safe diets alone, many wonder if they are safe to combine. This part of the book will discuss this. We will help you understand the ins, and outs of combining the diets.

All three diets share a similar theme which is restriction.

That may make you question two things. Is it possible to combine them? If so, are there extra benefits?

The answer to both is simple. Yes. It is possible to combine all three diets and get each of the benefits they offer.

Vegan keto is already a combination diet. Combining these will double the health benefits, as shown earlier. Both diets offer similar health benefits. Yet, there are a few which are unique to the individual diet. Combining any two diets will mean you can enjoy the benefits of both. This includes weight loss, lower risk of heart conditions, and neurological diseases. Then, as separate diets, they offer unique benefits. The vegan diet promotes life longevity. Whereas the keto diet offers benefits for epileptic patients. Then, by combining the diets, the participants reap the benefits of both.

For intermittent fasting, the diet method also offers similar health benefits. Yet, it also promotes other unique benefits. Such as cellular repair, autophagy, and reducing inflammation (79). Thus, combining all diets will allow the participant to enjoy all benefits.

Before combining all three of these diets, the body will need to adjust to the vegan keto first. The adapting stage is so the body can adjust to the new foods. It will need to adjust to the elimination of animal products. As well as the reduction of carbohydrates.

The longest part of the adapting stage may be getting over the keto flu. The keto flu signals that the body goes into shock. It does this as it tries to sync with the new low carbohydrate restrictions. Dieters will often experience nausea, weakness, irritability, headaches, and more according to studies.

By the time the body adjusts, vegan keto will feel like a lifestyle as opposed to a diet. Once the body completes the adapting stage, the body will feel more satisfied. Then, the next step is intermittent fasting.

Seeing as all diets pose efficacy, it is a great combination for greater health benefits.

Like all diets, there are pros and cons. Especially those which are a combination of diets. This chapter will assess the rights and wrongs. It will also prove, and display the extra health benefits. Use it as your guide for how to combine all three diets., and, be safe whilst doing so.

2

HOW DO DIETS WORK TOGETHER?

It is important to understand a bit more about how the three diets as a combination work together. Thus, there are three important things to cover. Number one is the benefits the participant can enjoy by practicing all three diets at once. The individual benefits of the diets are in the previous chapters. Thus, this section will cover the benefits of all three diets together. This will help you understand what benefits you may be able to enjoy.

Second, we will cover the risks of the combination diet. Covering this is essential for the participant's peace of mind, and knowledge. It will reveal the potential side effects. It will also cover who this combination is, and is not right for.

Last, we will address the pros, and cons of combining the diets. This will verify what is good, and bad about combining the three diets.

First, let's begin with the benefits the participant can enjoy:

3

BENEFITS OF PRACTICING ALL THREE DIETS TOGETHER

Y ou will already be aware of the health benefits of the three diets from previous chapters. So, this chapter will cover the benefits of practicing all three diets together.

There is not much research into this combination diet. Which means nobody can guarantee health benefits. Thus, these are the potential benefits most should experience.

Possibility to reach ketosis quicker

The keto diet promotes its ability to reach ketosis. This is where the body runs out of glucose and turns to fat as a fuel source. This encourages fat burning. Which is what makes the diet very popular for those seeking weight loss.

Intermittent fasting (IF) helps the body reach ketosis quicker. When the body is fasting, the energy balance switches from carbs to fat. Studies show that this is due to the body running low on glucose. Intermittent fasting promotes lowering insulin, and glycogen levels (80). This is the exact same premise as the keto diet. Hence, fasting alongside the vegan keto diet allows the body to reach ketosis quicker.

Once the body hits ketosis, the diet will be easier to sustain. Ketosis helps control hunger, which makes the participant eat less, and only when they need to. Not only will this make the diet easier, but it will also speed up weight loss.

Increased fat loss

The quicker the body reaches ketosis, the quicker the body will burn fat.

All dieting methods limit certain nutrients. Dietary limitations often result in fat loss. This is due to their increased metabolism. The increase in metabolic rate results in fat burning. Metabolism promotes thermogenesis, which is a process that utilizes stubborn stored fat (81).

The vegan keto diet does promote fat burning due to a decrease in carbohydrate intake. The substitute for plant-based proteins means the body has fewer carbs/glucose to burn. Thus, burns fat instead. This all results in fat loss.

Then, intermittent fasting is a method which is popular for its fat-burning abilities. Many studies reveal that the 16:8 IF method is most effective for fat burning. Participants of 16:8 can see 14% more fat loss than regular dieting (82).

Better mental clarity

When the body adapts to the vegan keto diet, it will manage to live off ketones. This is down to the fat fuel-burning used as a key source of energy for the brain, and the body. Fat is the most sustainable source of energy. The brain uses a lot of energy. Thus, is very beneficial for ulti-mate brain functioning.

The reason for the combination diet being better for mental clarity is due to ketosis. A normal diet involves high carbohydrates. Which means it relies on carbs for regular energy. Thus, when the body runs low on carbs, it will suffer, and feel weak.

But, if the body adapts to the lack of carbs, and runs off of fat fuel, it will always have a source of energy. This means your brain can run all the time instead of being energy-deprived (83).

More energy

Evidence shows that intermittent fasting methods can increase energy endurance (84). The same goes for the vegan keto diet. This is due to the calorie, and nutrient reductions because of timed eating periods. Athletes notice longer energy endurance during fasting periods. Their performance improves due to this.

To consume all essential nutrients, it is best to take supplements. This further will improve energy levels, and inhibit nutrient deficiencies.

Slower muscle loss

Studies reveal that intermittent fasting promotes slower muscle loss. Thus, helps preserve muscle mass. IF methods that allow a person to achieve autophagy increases muscle maintenance. Autophagy increases human growth hormones (HGH), which promotes muscle preservation (85).

This is beneficial alongside the keto diet, to increase fat loss and muscle gain. This is achievable due to the higher protein intake which the keto part of the diet requires. This combination diet is easy to sustain whilst being 100% vegan. This is as there are many plant-based protein substitutes.

A participant must ensure to eat the right amount of nutrients to sustain the vegan keto diet. Which will make intermittent fasting safe, and beneficial for muscle mass. This includes the correct intake of carbs, plant-based protein, and healthy fats on a daily basis. This will maximize results, and inhibit nutrient deficiencies.

There are many upsides to combining diets. Practicing the diets as one offers a multitude of incredible health benefits. Plus, it is easy to sustain being 100% vegan whilst doing so. There are now lots of plant-based options to choose from. Which makes it easier than ever to sustain a healthy balanced vegan keto diet. All whilst practicing intermittent fasting to optimize health benefits.

Although there are many benefits, there are a few risks you need to be aware of before combining the diets. For some, mild side effects may occur. For a few, the combination of the diets may pose health risks for existing conditions. Which, people should be aware of before practicing.

4

RISKS, PROS, AND CONS

L ike any diet, combination, or independent, there comes pros and cons. This may not be the case for everyone. But, these are the positives, and negatives that may occur for most participants.

Combining these diets is safe for most people. Yet, we must cover the cons of this combination diet. This is to cover and reflect upon the risks of the diet.

It is important to cover the pros and cons. So that people can know if the vegan keto and intermittent fasting diet are beneficial. Or, right for them.

Pros of Combining Vegan Keto with Intermittent Fasting

Appetite control

A typical diet involves a reasonable carbohydrate and protein intake. Which means a person consumes those foods to upkeep their energy.

Yet, low carb and plant-based protein diet can curb hunger easier.

Once the body adapts to the vegan keto diet, appetite is

easy to control. This is due to the body adjusting to the new foods. High fat and plant-based proteins take longer to digest. This means they fuel the body for longer due to the slow burn. Thus, the vegan keto part of the diet has proven to help control appetite, and curb hunger.

For intermittent fasting, this process is similar. The body adjusts to the new eating routine. Then, the body will soon only feel hungry during eating windows. Training your body into a new eating routine will help you eat less, and avoid unnecessary eating.

Quicker weight loss

Appetite control will be a major influence on weight loss. Eating less will guarantee a person to lose weight. With intermittent fasting involved, this will be the case.

The small, and cycled eating windows will help a person only eat during certain hours.

Also, this combination diet helps a person reach ketosis quicker. Ketosis promotes fat burning, which results in weight loss. Quicker fat-burning equals quicker weight loss.

Maximize ketosis

The vegan keto diet alone promotes fat burning. As it is a high-fat low carb diet, this means ketosis is easier to reach. This is due to the body consuming more fat than carbs, which means it will burn fat instead of glucose from carbs.

When fasting alongside the vegan keto diet, this will maximize ketosis. The periods without food will mean the body will run lower in carbs. During these hours the body can reach maximum ketosis. In some cases, the body will reach autophagy.

Helps maintain fat loss, and muscle mass

If the combination diet is done well, and a person sticks to the rules, this fat-burning will be easy to maintain.

Fat burning will continue as long as a person sticks to the right foods, and fasting routine.

This will improve body composition, which means muscle mass will be easy to maintain. With regular exercise, a person can maintain fat loss and muscle mass for as long as they wish. It all depends on how much effort a person puts into the diet. Effort equals maximize results.

Increases energy levels

High fat and plant-based protein diet promote slower digestion. Thus, the diet provides maximum fuel for the body. The longer the nutrients take to burn, the longer they will last as fuel.

Reduces the risk of heart disease

Both diets promote reducing the risk of heart disease. This includes lowering cholesterol, blood pressure, and preventing strokes, and heart attacks.

Risks of Combining Vegan Keto with Intermittent Fasting

Cannot guarantee the safety

There is not enough evidence to guarantee safety when combining these diets. It is up to the person to stick to the eating rules, and fasting routines. Then, if any side effects worsen or a person starts to feel ill, they must stop the diet. Seek medical advice to ensure you are not at risk of health complications.

May cause increased side effects from both diets

Studies suggest that a person may experience mild side effects with this diet. Thus, these side effects can worsen when combining both diets. This includes:

- Weakness

- Headaches
- Diarrhea
- Irritability
- Constipation
- Nausea
- Fatigue
- Poor concentration
- Muscle cramps
- Dizziness
- Trouble sleeping

If you experience any of these side effects for a long period of time (more than a few days) you must stop the diet, and seek advice.

Not easy/suitable for everyone

Both diets are not ideal for everyone. Thus, combining them can increase the people it is not ideal for. Those who should avoid this diet include:

- Anyone with a past or current eating disorder. This combination diet involves restricting foods and eating periods. This can worsen the disorder.
- Pregnant or breastfeeding women. There is not enough evidence to suggest fasting or a vegan keto diet is healthy for a baby's development.
- Women with amenorrhea. The combination excels in fat burning, and weight loss. These are both primary causes of amenorrhea. Thus, those with the condition should avoid this diet to prevent worsening the impact.

- Anyone with low blood pressure. Both diets can lower blood pressure. Thus, this combination diet can make blood pressure drop too low.
- Children or elder people. Children and elder people should avoid any food restrictive, and timed eating diets. It may stunt or slow children's growth. For elder people, it can intervene with current medications or conditions

Some may even try the diet for a while and get on well with it. Then, they might find it hard to maintain. Thus, it is not sustainable for everyone. As much as it is not suitable for anyone at high risk.

Seeing as this diet may not be for everyone, who is it ideal for?

5

WHO IS THIS COMBINATION DIET FOR?

First, this combination diet is ideal for anyone who is safe to try it. Those without health conditions or are not on the above list are safe to try the diet. Both men and women can be vegan keto, and reap equal benefits. The same goes for intermittent fasting. Thus, all people safe to try it can try it.

Then, anyone who is safe, and wishes to reap the diet's health benefits can partake in this diet.

People with a purpose, and goal will enjoy this diet. Anyone looking for quick weight loss, and fat burning will enjoy its quick ketosis gain.

For those looking to improve athletic performance will also enjoy this diet.

It is up to the person to ensure their own safety. Use the book as your guide for both diets, their rules, and plans. Then, use this section as your guide to help you understand how to combine the diets, and put it all together.

6

HOW TO PUT IT ALL TOGETHER

Combining the two diets is simple. Once you master the vegan keto diet, the next step is integrating intermittent fasting.

The main part of this diet is understanding what foods you can, and cannot eat. Intermittent fasting is not so much as diet, it restricts the times at which you eat. But, the vegan keto diet does involve food limitations. The reduction in carbohydrates is substituted with healthy fats and proteins. The animal products are substituted with non-dairy, animal-free plant-based substitutes. There is a strict, but extensive, food list to stick by for the vegan keto diet.

Vegan keto suggests you should get about 80 percent of your daily calories from fat. Then, 20 percent from plant-based protein, and 10 percent from carbohydrates.

On the vegan keto diet, fat is your friend. The substitution of fat allows the body to burn fat instead of glucose. This fat burning process is a metabolic state known as ketosis. Ketosis is beneficial for burning fat, and weight loss.

To consume a vegan keto diet you must eat lots of plant-based protein, low carb foods, and high-fat everything. The fat requirements are quite high. The fat you consume should always be healthy fats. These are best for the body and are those that promote health benefits.

Then, once you have planned your vegan keto diet, it is time to schedule in intermittent fasting. The timings and food cycles will depend on which method you have chosen. Let's say you have chosen the 16:8 time-restricted method. You should align your vegan keto meals in the 8-hour eating window. It is as simple as that.

Combining the two diets is not confusing. You need to eat vegan keto-based meals during the eating windows. Then you will be on a 100% vegan keto intermittent fasting diet. The in-depth food list for the vegan keto diet is in the previous chapter.

The following chapter will guide you through the meal planning process. There will be extensive knowledge of meal planning. As well as what foods to substitute for carbs and animal products. Plus, there will be weekly plans, daily routines, and many recipes to enjoy.

For any more queries or concerns about this combination diet, here is guidance for that:

E ven with the right knowledge, some may still have some questions. So, below are answers to the top questions about combining the diets:

Which has more benefits, vegan keto diet or intermittent fasting?

Both have very similar health benefits. The main reason for combining the two is for maximized benefits, and also to reach ketosis faster.

Neither is more beneficial than the other. That is up to the individual, and their health needs to decide. But, some may find intermittent fasting more achievable, and sustainable. This as it does not restrict any dietary nutrients. Those who struggle to cut carbs or animal products may find the vegan keto diet a challenge.

How long should you intermittent fasting on vegan keto?

Research suggests that intermittent fasting methods should change when on vegan keto. This is to ensure you do not encounter severe nutrient deficiency. You can take nutrient supplements alongside the diet. This is to prevent nutrient deficiency.

Some may also develop the refeeding syndrome. This is where the body sees a fatal shift in fluids, and electrolytes due to undernourishment. These shifts can cause detrimental effects to your health, and hormones.

What can I drink whilst intermittent fasting on vegan keto?

The diets promote the consumption of the same drinks intermittent fasting requires. This includes no-calorie drinks such as water, black coffee, or tea.

Can I exercise during fasting on vegan keto?

It is safe to exercise whilst fasting, even if choosing the extended 24-hour fast. As long as your body has enough energy, and hydration, it will cope if you exercise often.

Fasted cardiovascular exercise linked with excelled fat burning. As are vegan keto, and intermittent fasting. It is a good technique to use if your goal is to burn fat.

This combination diet is ideal for those looking to improve weight. As well as improving mental clarity, and energy endurance. The same for those who wish to reduce fat, and risk of heart disease. With the right knowledge, plan, and schedule anyone can enjoy the benefits of this diet. The vegan keto diet with intermittent fasting is safe. It is also simple, and sustainable with this as your guide.

PART VI

THE 4-STEP METHOD

« You will never change your life until you change something you do daily. The secret of your success is found in your daily routine. »

—John C. Maxwell

1

STEP 1 - CREATE YOUR NEW DAILY ROUTINE

Many may question why you need to create a daily routine in the first place. The answer is simple. Structure means success. Setting yourself daily tasks will help you stay on track. Being able to tick off a to-do list is helpful for most people.

Having structure to your day will also feel like your new eating habits are a lifestyle as opposed to a diet. It will help you establish your priorities. And, give you more willpower to complete everything on your list.

Setting a routine to suit your needs, and lifestyle is essential. What works for other people may not work for you. The key is to create a routine that helps you maximize your goals. It may take a little bit of trial, and error. But, you will get there with a few simple steps.

The first few steps may seem unnecessary. But believe us, they are the most important.

Make a list

First, you need to establish what you need to work on. For this, you need to be honest, positive, and visualize.

The list writing stage is where you need to be honest with yourself. Do not worry if your current diet is far from the vegan keto diet. From now is where change can happen. If your current eating lifestyle includes non-vegan, and non-keto foods, that is ok. Making a list of foods to need to get rid of to achieve the vegan keto diet will help you understand what is to come. This will be where you write a shopping list of the foods you will, and can eat on the vegan keto diet.

Next, you need to be positive. Being kind to yourself, and positive about the goals you aim to set will help place you in a positive mindset. Congratulate yourself for embarking on this journey. It is incredible that you are getting started. You should be proud of wanting to be a part of such an amazing eating journey.

The list you are creating needs to represent how you feel about your journey. It will need to encourage you, and motivate you to succeed. Let this part be about your personal development. The list should include the following. The foods you will be eating will most likely be first, as you have an understanding of this now. Then, you should decide when it is best to fast. This will be dependent on your current lifestyle, and routine. After this, make a list of your thoughts, and progressive ideas. This will help you visualize your goals. Visualization is key for seeing how, and if this eating lifestyle is sustainable for you. If you think it isn't before visualizing, then try this step. Without doing this, you may find it difficult to even try it out.

After you have made a list or a few, it is time to create a schedule.

Create a daily schedule

To fast right whilst being on the vegan keto diet, you will need a daily schedule. This will help you understand what to eat, and when to eat. It will also help you build a structure for your new eating lifestyle. This will make the diet seem less like a chore and more of a lifestyle.

Planning out your days will also allow you to motivate you to complete what you have written down. Schedules are fun to create, and even more satisfying to tick off. Enjoying what you have planned is key to success.

Make sure to be easy on yourself. Never overload your daily schedule. As this will make it unachievable, and not very enjoyable. Start with small goals, and build up the more you get to grips with the diet.

Breaking down days into time slots is ideal. Let's say you have a normal day of vegan keto and are intermittent fasting with the 16:8 method. It could look something like this:

- **8 am:** Start your day with affirmations. Give yourself a goal or a word for the day to stick to. This could be 'I Will achieve my weight loss goals of 62 kg by enjoying my new diet and sticking to my routine'. Or, it could be 'I will lose 10kg with this new diet. I will do exactly what I need to to be 100% vegan whilst on keto'. A daily affirmation will set the tone for the day, and help encourage you. You could do this in front of the mirror or even in bed. Doing it every day, 5 to 10 times in a row will help you stick to your convictions, and be self appreciative.

- **8:30 am:** Enjoy a calorie-free beverage. This can be water, black tea, or coffee. The intermittent fasting methods allow you to drink zero-calorie drinks throughout. A coffee or calming tea may be a good way to begin your day.
- **9 am:** Work begins. Work through the morning to take your mind off of eating, and to be productive. This will be a thing to tick off of your to-do list.
- **12 pm:** Break your fast. This could be with a late breakfast or lunch. Breaking your fast with a low carb meal is key. It is not only required for keto but also more beneficial when fasting. It prevents your blood sugar levels from spiking. Here, you could enjoy a tofu scramble, avocado, tomatoes, and spinach. You can add nuts, seeds, or high-fat oils on top. This will help you achieve the ultimate vegan keto meal.
- **1 pm:** Continue with work. Or, complete any chores. Whatever is on your to-do list, tick something off. Be productive. It is a good mindset to have.
- **4 pm:** Take a break, and have a snack. Vegan keto snacks can be fun, and perfect if you start feeling hungry. Enjoy some nuts, nut butter, berries, vegetables, or a low carb vegan protein shake or yogurt.
- **6 pm:** Move, move move. The early evening is an ideal time to exercise. You will have fuel from your breakfast/lunch, and snack. Exercising during this diet is safe, and maximizes the benefits. You can enjoy any type

of workout. From high-intensity interval training, cardio, or weight training.

- **7 pm:** Plan ahead. Write a tomorrows to-do list. Here is a good time to meal plan, plan your day, and more. Write down any thoughts or progress here too.
- **7:30 pm:** Last meal of the day. Dinner time should be right before you plan to fast. There are many meals you could enjoy. From Zucchini 'Pasta' to stir-fried veggies, and tofu. Make your meals fun, and flavorsome to please your needs.
- **8 pm:** Begin your fast. The evening is a great time to begin a fast. It allows your digestive system to rest overnight. Plus, it will seem like less time without food as for more of it, you will be asleep.

Creating a daily schedule every day is great for structure. It will help you to stay on track, and not give up. Planning your meals is a key part of the planning process.

Plan your meals, and your exercise

The key for the vegan keto diet is to eat well and eat right. Ensuring you get the right nutrients will inhibit nutrient deficiencies. Later in this chapter, you will discover 60 vegan keto recipes, which will help you with meal planning.

Combine the diet with exercise, and fun activities. It is safe to work out on the vegan keto diet as well as whilst intermittent fasting. You can even exercise whilst fasting to increase fat burning.

Making an exercise routine is as helpful as meal planning. This can be weekly planning to structure your workouts around your days. Three to five exercise days is healthy and gives balance.

As much as movement is beneficial, so is rest. Make sure you get enough sleep. Seven to eight hours per night is beneficial and provides the body with enough rest. Any diet and lifestyle need a good rest. Scheduling your sleep may seem odd. But, it will help you prioritize it over other non-essential things.

Check-in with yourself

Tracking progress, and staying on top of your daily schedule is a pathway to success. It will not only help you achieve your goals but will be a good way to see how far you have come. You can write down progress the traditional way. Or, there are many apps you can use to track your journey.

There are many online communities for the vegan keto, and intermittent fasting diets. Discussions will encourage you, and find like minded participants that are on the same journey.

These are some simple steps to help you achieve a successful daily routine. You will find a downloadable pdf to create your daily routine plan here with the password « veganketolifestyle » (https://fcer.org/vegan-keto-IF-book/).

2

STEP 2 - LET YOUR BODY ADAPT TO INTERMITTENT FASTING

I f you do not already do intermittent fasting, you will need to give your body time to adapt. This will not take long, but you will notice some changes during the adaptation stage.

Both diets will take around seven days for your body to adjust. Start with intermittent fasting. Try it for a week so your body can align with the new eating routine. If you need longer to feel comfortable, that is fine.

When your body has adjusted you will notice less fatigue, hunger, and irritability. This is where you start the adapting stage for the vegan keto diet. Again, take around a week to let your body adjust. You may experience the keto flu, which is where your body will be more tired, irritable, and weak than usual. The symptoms should decline after a week or ten days. When the symptoms wear off, this will signal that your body is adjusted.

If symptoms persist, it is best to stop the diet and seek professional advice. This diet will not be sustainable for everyone. But, you will not know until you try. There are no complications with this diet, only mild side effects.

. . .

If you do wish to continue, next are a few tips to help you stick to the diet.

3

STEP 3 - STICK TO YOUR CONVICTIONS

I n some circumstances, it can be difficult to stick to your convictions. But, with the right tips, you can have no trouble.

The hardest part of a diet like this is eating outside of your home. Social eating among friends in restaurants or at their homes may heighten some issues. But, there are easy ways around it.

Eating at restaurants or ordering a takeout

Many find it difficult to eat out. This is the cauliflower struggle. Most restaurants find cauliflower a good alternative to meat options. In fact, you do not need to live off of cauliflower. There are many amazing options to choose from. You just need to know about them.

The best cuisine for vegan keto is Asian food. Asian dishes are the most low carb options out there. Asian cuisines are often catering to vegan needs. There are lots of tofu, and veggie dishes to choose from. The best options are stir-fries or curries. For curries, choose coconut or tomato-based sauces. This could include chickpea curries, paneer tikkas, or onion fritters. Asian flavors will also spice up any diet. Do not give in to the cauliflower struggle. Asian foods are also often the lowest in carbs, and ideal for the vegan keto diet.

In Japanese restaurants, there are many options for vegan keto dieters. There are many smaller dishes that will satisfy the most. Such as Nasu dengaku, kaiso salads, and agedashi tofu.

For other restaurants, you can ask to skip the high carb or dairy products. For example, in Italian restaurants ask them to not add cheese. For restaurants that offer vegan burgers, you can go without the bun or substitute with lettuce.

Speaking of lettuce, make it fun. Swap any of your favorite high carb dishes for a lettuce base. Choose a vegan meal, and swap the carbs. Instead of rice, bread, and pasta have lettuce. That way you can still enjoy the yummy middle, just without the carbs.

If you are out for the day and need to eat out on the go, grain-free bars are a good option. There are many grain-free granola keto bars on the market to enjoy.

The great thing about dining with friends is that you can have an input in where you dine.

Dinner with friends

If you are the person with dietary requirements, always recommend places. This way you will be able to have leverage with the food choice. It is good to choose vegan places or those that cater to these needs.

If you are not going to a restaurant but plan to have a

social meal, invite your friends over. This will mean you will have full control over the foods, and you can align them to meet your requirements.

If you are going to a friend's house, offer to take a dish. This will create less fuss surrounding your dietary requirements. And, it will mean you have peace of mind with what you will eat.

Dealing with the keto flu

The keto flu is common for those first starting out. It is where your body will feel very tired, weak, and headaches can be frequent. This can make many people stop the diet altogether. It happens due to a drop or imbalance in potassium, and sodium. Both are electrolytes. Without them, your body will start to feel lackluster. This does not need to happen.

Sticking out the keto flu is simple if you know how to combat the symptoms. The best thing to do is to get your electrolytes back in check.

You can do this through a gallon of electrolyte fuelled liquid. To make this you need water. Then, add 2 teaspoons/55mg of naturacalm. This is a magnesium citrate powder. Follow this with 2 teaspoons of lite salt. Ensure the salt is an equal mix of potassium and sodium. If you wish, you can add flavor. Many like to use miodrops. These will give your liquid a fruity taste. There are many flavors to choose from. This combination will add enough electrolytes to your body to combat the keto flu.

For a quick liquid alternative, lemon water is great. Lemons are high in electrolytes which will give your body a quick boost. Ensuring you drink enough water is key for fatigue. Especially during the keto flu stage.

Also, grain-free keto bars are good for balancing blood

sugar levels. When you feel low on energy and weak, these can offer a good pick me up.

If you feel weak, this may indicate you are low in protein. A good suggestion is to have a pea protein shake. This will boost your carb intake, and balance blood sugar levels. Pea protein is the best option as most brands are vegan friendly.

Join an online community

Communities of like-minded individuals is a great way to feel part of a movement or team. Online communities can be encouraging, and very helpful.

These spaces allow you, and peers to share experiences. If you have any concerns or questions, communities are a great place to get advice. As the other people in the community will be on the same journey, it can give you peace of mind.

Also, be a better person, and share your tips. If you have found something new that works for you, then share it with others. It will help them, and in return, they might give you a top tip.

Join our online community **here** (http://www. facebook.com/groups/veganketodiet/)

The next step is discovering your new meal plan.

4

STEP 4 - DISCOVER YOUR INTERMITTENT FASTING & VEGAN KETO MEAL PLAN

G etting started with your new diet comes with a lot of new information. But, do not feel overwhelmed. When the right plan is in place, it will soon feel natural, and easy. Here are the top tips for structuring your meal planning process. Which will allow maximizing your benefits:

Download the full Meal Plan PDF with the last updated informations here with the password « veganketolifestyle »(https://fcer.org/vegan-keto-IF-book/). You will also find on this page a downloadable shopping list for each week.

If you are not fasting or choose a fasting method that allows an early breakfast

- **Do not eat after 8 pm**. It is best for your digestive system to rest overnight. With fasting, it is best to stop eating at a reasonable each day. This will mean your meal the following day is not too late. Studies have found that eating late means a person is eating excessive calories (86).

- **Lunchtime means lunch**. Do not snack or eat a small meal that will not sustain you. A meal full of healthy fats, and plant-based proteins will make you feel fuller, and give you energy for longer. Research has found that healthy fats contain medium-length triacylglycerols. These help the body feel fuller for longer (87). This is because they take longer to digest. They will fuel the body better than unhealthy fats. Bad fats contain short length triaclyglycerols. These do not sustain energy.

If you wish to eat breakfast, and are fasting

- **Eat an earlier dinner at 4 pm.** This will mean you can eat at 8am the following day. If you choose the 16:8 fast, you will need to fast for 16 hours. So, if you wish to eat an early breakfast you will need to stop eating early.

If you do not eat breakfast due to fasting

- **The lunch is at 12pm.** This can also be a late breakfast. But, it must be full of healthy fats, and protein to sustain you. Again, these will help sustain you. A high carb meal will cause blood sugar levels to spike. Also, carb intake is to be no greater than 45 grams per day. Thus, keep your carb intake as low as possible for all meals. This is because carbs can

come from many foods from fruits to
vegetables.

- **Have a snack around 4 pm.** This will
  provide you with energy, and reduce fatigue.
  Having a snack can also balance your blood
  sugar levels.
- **Dinner before 8 pm.** This will be the cut off
  time from eating. It also indicates the beginning
  of your fast. Most fasting techniques require an
  overnight fast that continues into the morning.
  Thus, stopping eating mid-evening will help
  you gut rest overnight.

Substitutions, and Finding Solutions For Allergies

If you have any allergies, please consult your nutritionist of
doctor for personalized medical advice before starting the
meal plan.

Or post a message to the community and we will give
you alternatives for you!

How to eat after the 4-week meal plan

The vegan keto diet with intermittent fasting is sustainable.
If you wish to continue the meal plan after the 4 weeks is
complete, you can.

If you decide not to be so strict with fasting but want to
stick to vegan keto, then follow the meal plans. Use the 60
recipes, in the following chapter, to find your favorite
meals. You could even repeat the meal plan for as many
weeks as you like.

To make it more fun, you could change the order of
the weeks. So long as you stick to the vegan keto meal
foods, you will successfully be on a vegan keto diet.

If you want some more meal plans, you can join the Facebook community where you, and others can share meal ideas.

The meal plans are more for the vegan keto part of this diet. This is due to intermittent fasting not requiring any specific foods. But, it specifies your mealtimes.

Thus, it is down to the individual which part of the diet they wish to sustain.

PART VII

THE 4-WEEK MEAL PLAN

With the help of:

Boon Get Up and Go - your personal dietician

∿

Monday

Lunch
arugula salad with avocado with olive oil
protein shake
Snack
almonds
power smoothie
coconut oil
Dinner
keto crackers
authentic guacamole
nuts pecans

Day 1: Calories 1,667 cal / Carbs 38 g (9%) / Protein 45
g (10%) / Fat 155 g (81%) / Fluid 4

∿

Tuesday

Lunch
overnight hemps
smooth peanut butter, no salt
Snack
arugula salad with avocado with olive oil
protein shake
Dinner
raw hazelnuts
blackberry & avocado smoothie

Day 2: Calories 1,640 cal / Carbs 46 g (11%) / Protein 63 g (15%) / Fat 138 g (74%) / Fluid 11

Wednesday

Lunch
chocolate bomb
protein shake
Snack
vegan keto bagels
almond butter, no salt
hemp seeds, raw
Dinner
mixed berry & coconut smoothie
hemp seeds, raw

Day 3: Calories 1,578 cal / Carbs 43 g (11%) / Protein 97 g (24%) / Fat 115 g (65%) / Fluid 1

Thursday

Lunch
big salad with olive oil
protein shake
Snack
keto pancake
homemade Nutella keto
chocolate bomb
Dinner
mixed berry & coconut smoothie
walnuts

Day 4: Calories 1,588 cal / Carbs 39 g (9%) / Protein 44
g (11%) / Fat 146 g (80%) / Fluid 1

Friday

Lunch
scrambled tofu
spinach with olive oil
fresh lemon juice
Snack
big salad with olive oil
hemp seeds, raw
Dinner
power smoothie
protein shake
smooth peanut butter, no salt

Day 5: Calories 1,512 cal / Carbs 37 g (10%) / Protein 72
g (19%) / Fat 119 g (71%) / Fluid 4

Saturday

Lunch
instant cereal
hemp seeds, raw
100% natural zero-calorie sweetener by stevia
flaxseed oil
Snack
strawberry spinach salad with olive oil
chia seeds
Dinner
blueberry & cashew smoothie
nuts pecans
protein shake

Day 6: Calories 1,681 cal / Carbs 40 g (9%) / Protein 48
g (11%) / Fat 153 g (80%) / Fluid 2

Sunday

Lunch
vegan keto bagels
homemade nutella keto
hemp seeds, raw
Snack
vegan cream cheese
keto crackers
walnuts (raw)
Dinner

veggie smoothie
hemp seeds, raw
flaxseed oil

Day 7: Calories 1,637 cal / Carbs 37 g (9%) / Protein 51 g (12%) / Fat 147 g (79%) / Fluid 2

∽

Monday

Lunch
fried bok choy with olive oil
healing cleanse protein shake
Snack
raw mixed nuts
hemp seeds, raw
natural peanut butter
Dinner
tofu stir fry
flaxseed oil

Day 1: Calories 1,641 cal / Carbs 39 g (9%) / Protein 56
g (13%) / Fat 146 g (78%) / Fluid 14

∽

Tuesday

Lunch
nuts pecans
coconut butter
healing cleanse protein shake
Snack
vegan keto bagels with vegan cream cheese
almonds hemp seeds, raw
Dinner
zucchini meatballs
flaxseed oil

Day 2: Calories 1,593 cal / Carbs 41 g (10%) / Protein 39 g (10%) / Fat 145 g (80%) / Fluid 7

Wednesday

Lunch
mixed berry & coconut smoothie
walnuts
protein shake
Snack
chia pudding
chocolate bomb
Dinner
raw walnut taco "meat" with olive oil

Day 3: Calories 1,578 cal / Carbs 39 g (9%) / Protein 48 g (12%) / Fat 145 g (79%) / Fluid 0

Thursday

Lunch
vegan protein shake
peanut butter energy balls
Snack
hemp seeds, raw
natural peanut butter
Dinner
tempeh bacon with flaxseed oil

Day 4: Calories 1,685 cal / Carbs 39 g (9%) / Protein 90 g (21%) / Fat 128 g (70%) / Fluid 3

Friday

Lunch
power smoothie
flaxseed oil
protein shake
Snack
keto crackers
almond butter, no salt
Dinner
tempeh bacon with olive oil

Day 5: Calories 1,676 cal / Carbs 41 g (10%) / Protein 54 g (13%) / Fat 149 g (77%) / Fluid 2

Saturday

Lunch

blueberry & cashew smoothie

almonds

flaxseed oil

Snack

peanut butter energy balls

hemp seeds, raw

Dinner

bunless veggie burgers with avocado and olive oil

Day 6: Calories 1,657 cal / Carbs 37 g (9%) / Protein 54 g (13%) / Fat 150 g (78%) / Fluid 3

Sunday

Lunch

healing cleanse protein shake

hemp seeds, raw

Snack

chocolate bomb

almonds

Dinner

marinated baked tempeh with olive oil

Day 7: Calories 1,610 cal / Carbs 40 g (10%) / Protein 60 g (14%) / Fat 140 g (76%) / Fluid 14

WEEK THREE

Monday

Lunch
blueberry & cashew smoothie
walnuts
hemp seeds, raw
Snack
chocolate bomb
Dinner
garlic Tamarii tempeh and broccoli with olive oil

Day 1: Calories 1,622 cal / Carbs 38 g (9%) / Protein 44 g (11%) / Fat 147 g (80%) / Fluid 2

Tuesday

Lunch
vegan protein shake
keto crackers
Snack
chocolate bomb
mixed nuts
Dinner
chopped spinach salad
flaxseed oil

Day 2: Calories 1,697 cal / Carbs 39 g (9%) / Protein 54 g (13%) / Fat 142 g (78%) / Fluid 7

~

Wednesday

Lunch
mixed berry & coconut smoothie
almonds
protein shake
Snack
homemade nutella keto
keto crackers
Dinner
tofu & veggies in peanut sauce with olive oil

Day 3: Calories 1,628 cal / Carbs 39 g (9%) / Protein 52 g (12%) / Fat 145 g (79%) / Fluid 3

~

Thursday

Lunch
power smoothie
flaxseed oil
protein shake
Snack
keto crackers
authentic guacamole
olive oil
Dinner
tofu stir fry with olive oil

Day 4: Calories 1,654 cal / Carbs 40 g (9%) / Protein 63 g (15%) / Fat 144 g (76%) / Fluid 13

Friday

Lunch
healing cleanse protein shake
walnuts
Snack
walnut red pepper dip
keto crackers
flaxseed oil
Dinner
marinated baked tempeh with olive oil

Day 5: Calories 1,691 cal / Carbs 39 g (9%) / Protein 72 g (16%) / Fat 144 g (75%) / Fluid 10

Saturday

Lunch
mixed berry & coconut smoothie
peanut butter energy balls
flaxseed oil
Snack
peanut butter energy balls
hemp seeds, raw
Dinner
garlic Tamarii tempeh and broccoli with olive oil

Day 6: Calories 1,620 cal / Carbs 39 g (9%) / Protein 38 g (9%) / Fat 148 g (82%) / Fluid 2

Sunday

Lunch
vegan protein shake
keto crackers
Snack
chocolate bomb
mixed nuts
Dinner
chopped spinach salad
flaxseed oil

Day 7: Calories 1,697 cal / Carbs 39 g (9%) / Protein 54 g (13%) / Fat 142 g (78%) / Fluid 7

WEEK FOUR

~

Monday

Lunch
veggie smoothie
flaxseed oil
protein shake
Snack
vegan keto bagels
walnut red pepper dip
Dinner
chopped spinach salad with olive oil

Day 1: Calories 1,610 cal / Carbs 35 g (8%) / Protein 45
g (11%) / Fat 150 g (81%) / Fluid 6

~

Tuesday

Lunch
healing cleanse protein shake
big salad with olive oil
Snack
chocolate bomb
walnuts
Dinner
scrambled tofu
vegan keto bagels with vegan cream cheese
flaxseed oil

Day 2: Calories 1,550 cal / Carbs 40 g (10%) / Protein 52 g (13%) / Fat 134 g (77%) / Fluid 8

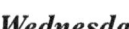

Wednesday

Lunch
blueberry & cashew smoothie 1
protein shake
Snack
vegan keto bagels
homemade nutella keto
almonds
Dinner
arugula salad with avocado and olive oil

Day 3: Calories 1,615 cal / Carbs 38 g (9%) / Protein 43 g (10%) / Fat 147 g (81%) / Fluid 4

Thursday

Lunch
hemp seeds, raw
healing cleanse protein shake

Snack
chocolate bomb
almonds
coconut oil

Dinner
tempeh bacon with olive oil

Day 4: Calories 1,657 cal / Carbs 40 g (9%) / Protein 63 g (15%) / Fat 145 g (76%) / Fluid 9

Friday

Lunch
power smoothie
almonds
protein shake

Snack
tempeh bacon
big salad with olive oil

Dinner
fried bok choy
raw walnut taco "meat"
olive oil

Day 5: Calories 1,649 cal / Carbs 40 g (9%) / Protein 57 g (13%) / Fat 147 g (78%) / Fluid 3

Saturday

Lunch
blackberry & avocado smoothie
chia pudding
hemp seeds, raw
coconut oil
Snack
chocolate bomb
protein shake
Dinner
avocado tahini salad with olive oil

Day 6: Calories 1,594 cal / Carbs 37 g (9%) / Protein 53 g (13%) / Fat 143 g (78%) / Fluid 6

Sunday

Lunch
vegan protein shake
Snack
keto pancake
homemade nutella keto
Dinner
marinated baked tempeh
cucumber with olive oil

Day 7: Calories 1,654 cal / Carbs 40 g (10%) / Protein 61 g (15%) / Fat 133 g (75%) / Fluid 8

PART VIII

37 KETO VEGAN RECIPES

1

SAVOURY

~

Arugula salad with avocado

Ingredients

- olive oil 3 Tbsp
- avocados 1/4 avocado

Nutrition Totals: Calories 447 / Carbs 6g / Protein 2g / Fat 48g / Fluid 2 fl oz

Instructions

1. Chop the avocado tomato and red onion as desire.
2. Add to a bowl with the regular.
3. Add olive oil, lemon juice, salt, and pepper as desire.
4. Mix and serve.

Keto crackers

Ingredients

- seeds flaxseed 150 gm
- chia seeds 3 Tbsp
- drinking water 1 Cup(s)
- hemp hearts raw shelled 3 Tbsp
- sunflower seeds (raw, shelled) 3 tablespoon(s)
- sesame seeds 8 tsp
- herbs italian seasoning by schwartz 20 gram

Nutrition Totals: Calories 1885 / Carbs 96g / Protein 74g / Fat 141g / Fluid 8 fl oz

Instructions *(10 serving)*

1. Preheat the oven to 200F. Line baking sheet with a parchment paper.
2. Combine the flaxseeds and chia seeds with the water

in a mixing bowl. Mix well and ensure everything has been coated with the water. Let sit for 20 minutes.

3. Add the rest of the ingredients and mix well.

4. Spread the mixture as thinly as possible onto the parchment paper-lined baking tray. Use the back of a spoon or spatula to smooth out the mixture so it is evenly spread, making sure there are no holes.

5. Cut the crackers with knife for even squares.

6. Bake for 1 1/2 hours and then flip the cracker mixture over using a spatula. It should stay together, but still be a bit flexible at this point. I sometimes find placing a new sheet of parchment paper on the tray and flipping the mixture onto that works best. Bake for another 1 1/2 hours.

7. Once the crackers have baked for a total of 3 hours, turn the oven off but let the crackers stay in the warmed oven to cook further for another 20 minutes.

8. Remove from oven and let crackers cool.

Store in a sealed container up to 7 days.

Authentic guacamole

Ingredients

- avocados 1/2 avocado
- serrano peppers 1/4 Cup(s)
- onions 1/4 cuplimes 1 oz
- cilantro leaves raw, coriander 2 tsp

Nutrition Totals: Calories 189 / Carbs 16g / Protein 3g / Fat 15g / Fluid 4 fl oz

Instructions (1 serving)

1. Mash the onion, chile, 1/2 cilantro, and salt to a paste in a « molcajete ».

2. With a knife, score the flesh in the avocado halves in a crosshatch pattern, and then scoop into the bowl.

3. Toss it, then mash coarsely with a fork and add all the cilantro.

4. Season it to taste with lime juice, and add salt and chile.

~

Vegan keto bagels

Ingredients

- ground flax seeds 1/4 Cup(s)
- psyllium husk 4 Tbsp
- baking powder 1 teaspoon(s)
- seeds sesame butter paste 1/2 Cup(s)
- drinking water 1 Cup(s)
- sea salt 1/4 teaspoon(s)

Nutrition Totals: Calories 958 / Carbs 54g / Protein 28g / Fat 75g / Fluid 8 fl oz

. . .

Instructions (6 servings)

1. Preheat oven to 375F.
2. To a food processor, add psyllium husk, ground flax seeds, baking powder, and salt, and whisk until thoroughly combined
3. Add the water to the tahini, and whisk until combined.
4. Stir the dry ingredients into the wet, and then knead to form the dough.
5. Form patties by hand that are about 4" in diameter, and 1/4" thick.
6. Lay on your baking tray and cut a small circle from the middle of each round
7. Add the sesame seeds.
8. Bake for 45 minutes, until it become golden brown.

Big salad

Ingredients

- salads organic spring mix by earthbound farm 2 Cup(s)
- radishes 1/2 cup
- black pepper 1/4 tsp
- cherry tomatoes 10 tomatoes

Nutrition Totals: Calories 197 / Carbs 17g / Protein 4g / Fat 14g / Fluid 3 fl oz

Instructions (1 serving)

1. Chop the veggies as desire.
2. Add to a bowl.
3. Add seasonings and olive oil and serve.

Scrambled tofu

Ingredients

- firm tofu by nasoya 250 gram
- spices turmeric ground 1/4 tsp
- original unsweetened pure almond milk by silk 140 mL

Nutrition Totals: Calories 241 / Carbs 7g / Protein 23g / Fat 11g / Fluid 0 fl oz

Instructions

1. In a large, non-stick frying pan, break the tofu into bite-sized pieces.
2. Over medium heat, stir in turmeric and the

nutritional yeast, until it is well combined. Cook for 6 minutes.

3. Add the almond milk and simmer for an 11 minutes more, stir occasionally until the tofu becomes creamy.
4. Adding salt and black pepper is optional.

Strawberry spinach salad

Ingredients

- olive oil 3 Tbsp
- spinach 3 Cup(s)

Nutrition Totals: Calories 406 / Carbs 10g / Protein 3g / Fat 41g / Fluid 5 fl oz

Instructions (1 serving)

1. Broil or roast turkey breast thoroughly.
2. In a medium size bowl, whisk together the vinegar, and the olive oil.
3. In a large size bowl, mix the spinach. strawberries Combine chopped turkey breast.
4. Pour dressing over salad, and toss. Refrigerate 10 to 15 minutes before serving.

Vegan cream cheese

Ingredients

- cashews (raw) 1 1/2 cup(s)
- coconut cream by savoy 1/2 Cup(s)
- onion powder 1 tsp

Nutrition Totals: Calories 2042 / Carbs 104g / Protein 61g / Fat 154g / Fluid 2 fl oz

Instructions

1. Soak cashews in hot water for 1 hour.
2. Add the soaked cashews (drained), coconut cream, lemon juice, salt, white vinegar, and onion powder into the food processor and blend.
3. Stop regularly, scrape down sides, stir and continue until it become very smooth.
4. Transfer the mix into a bowl, add in the dill, and stir.
5. Keep it in a fridge overnight and enjoy!

Fried bok choy

Ingredients

- basil (fresh) 1 tablespoon(s)
- black pepper (ground) 1/4 teaspoon(s)
- coconut oil 2 tablespoons
- soy sauce made from Tamarii 5 tsp
- fresh lemon juice 2 Tbsp

Nutrition Totals: Calories 301 / Carbs 8g / Protein 6g / Fat 29g / Fluid 2 fl oz

Instructions (1 serving)

1. Put the coconut oil in a large skillet on medium heat.
2. Add Tamarii and bok choy, cook for 5 minutes until greens become limp through heat and stalks are crispy.
3. Add some seasoning, and enjoy.

Tofu stir fry

Ingredients

- broccoli 1/2 cup

- tofu, extra firm 200 gm
- coconut oil 1 tablespoons
- red peppers 1/2 cup
- mushrooms 1 cup

Nutrition Totals: Calories 356 / Carbs 14g / Protein 24g / Fat 26g / Fluid 11 fl oz

Instructions (1 serving)
Mix all ingredients into a skillet and saute until almost tender.

~

Zucchini meatballs

Ingredients

- shredded zucchini 1 Cup(s)
- sea salt 1/4 teaspoon(s)
- walnuts chopped by 365 1 Cup(s)
- psyllium husk 1 Tbsp
- Italian seasoning by tampico 3 tsp

Nutrition Totals: Calories 241 / Carbs 14g / Protein 6g / Fat 18g / Fluid 0 fl oz

. . .

Instructions (1 serving)

1. Preheat your oven to 350°F (177°C) and line a baking sheet with parchment paper.
2. In a medium bowl, stir together chopped walnuts, grated zucchini, and salt.
3. Let it sit for about four minutes.
4. Add seasoning and psyllium, then stir until combined.
5. Let it sit for four minutes more.
6. With your hands, form some golfball-sized balls and place them on the baking tray.
7. Bake for 35 min, the goal is to have the zucchini balls a little bit brown on the outside and firm when you touch.

Raw walnut taco "meat"

Ingredients

- garlic cloves peeled by spice world 4 serving
- paprika 2 tsp
- salt 1/4 tsp
- 100% natural zero calorie sweetener by stevia in the raw 2 packet

Nutrition Totals:

Calories 2473 / Carbs 79g / Protein 61g / Fat 237g / Fluid 2 fl oz

Instructions (6 Servings)

1. Add sun-dried tomatoes to a small bowl and cover with warm water. Set aside for 5 minutes.
2. Add walnuts in the bowl of the food processor, and pulse into a fine meal. Then transfer walnuts to a mid-size bowl and set aside.
3. Drain the sundried tomatoes (reserve all the water in a bowl to add it back to the sauce later) and add to the food processor's bowl.
4. Add sea salt, smoked paprika, garlic, cumin, coconut sugar, habaneros, chili powder, and nutritional yeast (option) and blend it until it forms a smooth paste.
5. Add 1 tablespoon of reserved water at a time until it forms a thick sauce.
6. Taste it and adjust the flavor if needed.
7. Add the all mixture to walnuts and stir it until combined.
8. Enjoy it!

Tempeh bacon

Ingredients

- olive oil 1 tbsp

- soy sauce made from Tamarii 30 mL
- liquid smoke by colgin 1/2 tsp
- black pepper 1/4 tsp
- syrup, sugar-free 1 Tbsp
- sea salt 1/2 teaspoon(s)
- garlic powder 1/2 tsp

Nutrition Totals: Calories 372 / Carbs 17g / Protein 25g / Fat 26g / Fluid 3 fl oz

Instructions (1 Servings)

1. Cut tempeh in quarter (5 mm) thick slices.
2. Add the tempeh to a grease frying pan, over medium heat.
3. Cook for 4 minutes on each side until it become crispy-tender and brown.
4. Add water (1 tbsp) to the pan and stir.
5. Add all the ingredients: syrup, soy sauce, liquid smoke, black pepper, garlic, and stir until tempeh is uniformly covered.
6. Let it become brown for around 3 minutes, and enjoy.

Bunless veggie burgers with avocado

Ingredients

- meat free burgers, vegan 14 oz
- cucumber, peeled 1 large
- onions 1/2 Cup(s)

Nutrition Totals: Calories 624 / Carbs 57g / Protein 78g / Fat 18g / Fluid 13 fl oz

Instructions (4 Servings)

1. In a medium-sized bowl, stir avocados, cucumber, lemon juice, green onion and salt.
2. Arrange a lettuce leaf on each of 4 plates.
3. Place a vegetable burger on each leaf; top with tomato and cucumber slices, and avocado mixture.

Marinated baked tempeh

Ingredients

- tempeh 200 gm
- 100% natural zero calorie sweetener by stevia in the raw 1 packet
- black pepper 1/4 tsp

Nutrition Totals: Calories 570 / Carbs 29g / Protein 45g / Fat 35g / Fluid 6 fl oz

Instructions (1 serving)

1. After cutting the tempeh into little cubes, steam it for 9 to 11 minutes.
2. In a small bowl, mix together the stevia, olive oil, tamarii, vinegar, and pepper.
3. Add the tempeh in a dish and pour the marinade on top to coat. Let it marinate for 35 minutes.
4. Preheat the oven to 425°F.
5. Line baking sheet and parchment paper.
6. Place the cubes on the baking sheet, keep the excess of marinade.
7. Bake for 12 minutes.
8. Remove the tempeh from the oven and add marinade on the cubes
9. Bake 12 more minutes.
10. Enjoy!

Garlic tamarii tempeh and broccoli

Ingredients

- nutritional yeast flakes super food by now 1/4 Cup(s)
- tempeh 150 gm
- sweet drops liquid stevia by sweet leaf 5 drops
- soy sauce made from tamari 30 gm

Nutrition Totals: Calories 825 / Carbs 43g / Protein 34g / Fat 48g / Fluid 7 fl oz

Instructions (2 Servings)

1. Cut the tempeh into 1/4 inch strips.
2. In a large skillet over medium-low heat brown the tempeh strips with a little oil, or cooking spray, adding more oil, as necessary to keep the pan from drying out.
3. Once tempeh is golden brown in color, add tamarii, stevia and nutritional yeast and mix to coat tempeh.
4. Add broccoli and garlic to pan. Simmer mixture for about 10 minutes, turning occasionally.
5. Remove from heat once broccoli is tender-crisp and bright in color,
6. Serve.

Chopped spinach salad

Ingredients

- olive oil 1 Tbsp
- black pepper 1 tsp
- spinach 3 Cup(s)
- walnuts 1/4 cup

Nutrition Totals: Calories 503 / Carbs 19g / Protein 9g / Fat 48g / Fluid 6 fl oz

Instructions

1. Chop the avocado.
2. Combine all the ingredients and serve.

Tofu & veggies in peanut sauce

Ingredients

- broccoli 1 cup
- smooth peanut butter, no salt 2 Tbsp
- tofu, extra firm 8 oz
- natural stevia sweetener by sweetleaf 1 packet

Nutrition Totals: Calories 459 / Carbs 22g / Protein 37g / Fat 30g / Fluid 12 fl oz

Instructions (1 serving)

1. Heat oil in a large skillet or wok over medium-high heat. Sauté broccoli, , mushrooms and tofu for 5 minutes.
2. In a small bowl combine peanut butter, 1/4 C hot water, vinegar, stevia& tamarii.
3. Pour over vegetables and tofu. Simmer for 3 to 5 minutes, or until vegetables are tender crisp.

Walnut red pepper dip

Ingredients

- shelled walnuts by safeway 2 Cup(s)
- fire roasted red peppers by trader joe's 1 1/2 Cup(s)
- olive oil 2 Tbsp
- cumin ground 1/2 tsp

Nutrition Totals: Calories 1765 / Carbs 51g / Protein 35g / Fat 171g / Fluid 1 fl oz

Instructions

1. In a food processor, pulse walnuts, cumin, and salt until walnuts are finely ground.
2. Add peppers, garlic, olive oil, and lemon juice.
3. Whirl until smooth.

Cauliflower coconut mash

Ingredients

- coconut milk light by blue dragon 1/4 Cup(s)
- sea salt fine crystals by trader joe's 1/8 tsp
- peppers ground black by schwartz 1/8 gram

Nutrition Totals: Calories 341 / Carbs 37g / Protein 16g / Fat 19g / Fluid 18 fl oz

Instructions (2 servings)

1. Add all ingredients into a pot and bring to boil on medium heat Reduce to low and cover with a lid.
2. Simmer for 15 mins and then remove from heat
3. Pulse in a blender or a food processor until smooth.

4. Add a tablespoon of water if it's too thick during mixing.
5. You can also mash it with a fork if you don't have a blender.

Avocado tahini salad

Ingredients

- avocados 1/2 avocado
- organics baby spring mixed greens 3 Cup(s)
- fresh lemon juice 1 Tbsp

Nutrition Totals: Calories 282 / Carbs 19g / Protein 7g / Fat 23g / Fluid 4 fl oz

Instructions

1. Chop the avocado and the cucumber as desire, add to a bowl with the spring mix.
2. Mix the tahini (sesame butter) with lemon juice a little bit water salt and pepper (optional).
3. Mix together and serve.

2

SMOOTHIE

∾

Power smoothie

Ingredients

- strawberries (fr oz en) 1/4 cup(s)
- almond milk (unsweetened) 1 1/2 cup(s)
- almond butter (unsweetened) 1 2/3 tablespoon(s)
- sea salt
- 1/4 teaspoon(s)

Nutrition Totals: Calories 427 / Carbs 17g / Protein 9g / Fat 37g / Fluid 0 fl oz

. . .

Instructions

mix all the ingredients and serve

❧

Blackberry & avocado smoothie

Ingredients

- avocados 1/4 avocado
- cilantro leaves raw, coriander 1 tsp
- drinking water 3/4 Cup(s)

Nutrition Totals: Calories 129 / Carbs 9g / Protein 3g / Fat 10g / Fluid 9 fl oz

Instructions

1. Add water into blender and then add ingredients.
2. Blend.
3. Add ice if desired.

❧

Mixed berry & coconut smoothie

Ingredients

- kale (raw) 1/2 cup(s)
- almond butter (unsweetened) 1 tablespoon(s)
- coconut milk (unsweetened, canned) 1/2 cup(s)
- coconut butter by kerala 1 Tbsp

Nutrition Totals: Calories 482 / Carbs 18g / Protein 9g / Fat 44g / Fluid 0 fl oz

Instructions

1. Add the kale to a blender.
2. Pour 1/2 cups coconut milk and 2/3 cups almond milk into the blender.
3. Blend until large pieces of green are no longer visible in the blender.
4. Add the blueberries to the blender.
5. Add 1 tablespoon coconut butter, 1 tablespoon almond butter, and 1/4 teaspoon salt to the blender.
6. Blend until smooth, about 30 to 45 seconds.
7. pour into a tall glass and serve.

Blueberry & cashew smoothie

Ingredients

- cashews (raw) 1/4 cup(s)
- almond milk (unsweetened) 1 1/4 cup(s)
- pure vanilla extract 2 teaspoon(s)

Nutrition Totals: Calories 254 / Carbs 11g / Protein 8g / Fat 20g / Fluid 0 fl oz

Instructions (1 serving)
Mix all the ingredients and serve.

∽

Veggie smoothie

Ingredients

- ginger root 1/2 tsp
- celery 1 small stalk
- cucumber 1/4 cucumber
- spices turmeric ground 1/4 tsp
- original unsweetened almond milk breeze by blue diamond 250 mL

Nutrition Totals: Calories 342 / Carbs 15g / Protein 12g / Fat 29g / Fluid 3 fl oz

. . .

Instructions

Add ingredients to blender with handful of ice cubes, blend and drink immediately.

❧

Mixed berry & coconut smoothie

Ingredients

- kale (raw) 1/2 cup(s)
- almond butter (unsweetened) 1 tablespoon(s)
- coconut milk (unsweetened, canned) 1/2 cup(s)
- coconut butter by kerala 1 Tbsp

Nutrition Totals: Calories 482 / Carbs 18g / Protein 9g / Fat 44g / Fluid 0 fl oz

Instructions

1. Add the kale to a blender.
2. Pour 1/2 cups coconut milk and 2/3 cups almond milk into the blender.
3. Blend until large pieces of green are no longer visible in the blender.
4. Add the blueberries to the blender.
5. Add 1 tablespoon coconut butter, 1 tablespoon

almond butter, and 1/4 teaspoon salt to the blender.

6. Blend until smooth, about 30 to 45 seconds.
7. Pour into a tall glass and serve.

3

PROTEIN SHAKE

∾

Vegan Protein shake

Ingredients

- blueberries 1/2 cups
- coconut water 1/2 Cup(s)
- natural plant-based protein powder chocolate 1 scoop

Nutrition Totals: Calories 470 / Carbs 14g / Protein 36g / Fat 21g / Fluid 4 fl oz

Instructions

Mix all ingredient together in a blender and blend to desired consistency and enjoy great for before or after a workout.

Healing cleanse protein shake

Ingredients

- celery 1 medium stalk
- parsley 4 sprigs
- ginger root 1 slices (1" dia)
- drinking water 1 Cup(s)
- vanilla Protein powder 1 scoop

Nutrition Totals: Calories 240 / Carbs 19g / Protein 29g / Fat 6g / Fluid 13 fl oz

Instructions (1 serving)

Combine water and ingredients into blender and blend. Enjoy!

protein shake

Ingredients

- water 400ml
- natural plant-based protein powder chocolate or vanilla 1 scoop

Nutrition Totals: Calories 120 / Carbs 4g / Protein 20g / Fat 2,5g / Fluid 13 fl oz

Instructions

Mix water with protein powder in a shake. Shake it, drink it!

4

SWEET

Chocolate bomb

Ingredients

- almond butter, no salt 1/2 Cup(s)
- cocoa dry powder unsweetened 1/4 Cup(s)
- 100% natural zero calorie sweetener by stevia in the raw 1 packet

Nutrition Totals: Calories 1355 / Carbs 38g / Protein 31g / Fat 130g / Fluid 0 fl oz

Instructions (6 Servings)

1. Stir all ingredients together until smooth. If too dry, add additional coconut oil if needed.
2. Pour into a small container, ice cube trays, candy molds.
3. Freeze to set. Because coconut oil softens when warm, it's best to store these in the freezer.

Keto pancake

Ingredients

- almond butter, no salt 2 Tbsp
- ground flaxseed 1 Tbsp
- baking powder 1/2 teaspoon(s)
- original unsweetened pure almond milk by silk 1/4 Cup(s)
- coconut flour 1 tablespoon(s)
- 100% natural zero calorie sweetener by stevia in the raw 2 packet

Nutrition Totals: Calories 313 / Carbs 18g / Protein 11g / Fat 26g / Fluid 0 fl oz

Instructions

- Heat your frying pan on low medium heat, with a little grease or cooking spray.
- In a small dish, combine almond butter and almond milk.
- In another dish, combine the dry ingredients until well blended.
- Combine wet and dry ingredients, and stir until thoroughly mixed.
- Let this sit for 5 minutes. make 3-4 pancakes with this amount.
- Cook for about 4-5 minutes, until the pancake flips easily.
- When golden on the underside, flip and cook for another 2-3 minutes until done.

Homemade nutella keto

Ingredients

- raw hazelnuts by basse 300 gram
- cocoa dry powder unsweetened 1/4 Cup(s)

Nutrition Totals: Calories 2189 / Carbs 62g / Protein 4g / Fat 211g / Fluid 0 fl oz

Instructions (10 Servings)

1. Preheat the oven to 350F/180C.
2. Spread out raw hazelnuts on a baking tray with parchment paper and roast for around 10 minutes, until golden brown.
3. Remove the skins from the hazelnuts and set aside.
4. Add the hazelnuts to a food processor, and pulse until it becomes a smooth paste, make sure to scrape down the side so the mixture will all combine.
5. Add the rest of your ingredients and blend until smooth and creamy.

If the Nutella is too thick, add a little extra coconut oil.

Instant cereal

Ingredients

- coconut flour 6 tablespoon(s)
- sea salt 1/8 teaspoon(s)
- original unsweetened pure almond milk by silk 270 gram
- 100% natural zero calorie sweetener by stevia in the raw 2 packet
- chopped walnuts by diamond of California 1/4 Cup(s)

Nutrition Totals: Calories 448 / Carbs 51g / Protein 14g / Fat 24g / Fluid 3 fl oz

Instructions

- Stir together all ingredients in a bowl. It may seem thin at first, but you have to keep stirring until the coconut flour absorbs all the liquid and it thickens.
- Add more milk if a thinner porridge is preferred.
- Top with blueberries and cashews.
- Eat cold, or heat if desired.

Chia pudding

Ingredients

- coconut milk beverage, unsweetened 1/4 Cup(s)
- original unsweetened pure almond milk by silk 1/4 Cup(s)
- 100% natural zero calorie sweetener by stevia in the raw 2 packet

Nutrition Totals: Calories 351 / Carbs 34g / Protein 11g / Fat 22g / Fluid 0 fl oz

. . .

Instructions (2 servings)

1. Mix the chia seeds, coconut milk, almond milk, cacao powder, and stevia 2. If you prefer a smoother texture, use ground chia seed.
2. Let it sit for at least 10-15 minutes, ideally overnight in the fridge.
3. Serve, store up to 4 days in the refrigerator.

Peanut butter energy balls

Ingredients

- steeves maples 1 1/2 tablespoons
- coconut flour 4 tablespoon(s)

Nutrition Totals: Calories 861 / Carbs 45g / Protein 36g / Fat 65g / Fluid 0 fl oz

Instructions (3 Servings- 15 balls)

1. Add peanut butter, coconut flour, and keto maple syrup.
2. Stir with a fork until well mixed. Then, use a silicone spatula to fold until well incorporated and thickened.
3. Using a small or medium cookie scoop, scoop

and drop peanut butter balls onto baking sheet with parchment paper spaced evenly apart.

Overnight hemps

Ingredients

- coconut milk, canned, full-Fat sprouts organic 2/3 cups
- chia seeds 1 Tbsp
- vanilla extract 1/2 tsp

Nutrition Totals: Calories 833 / Carbs 21g / Protein 32g / Fat 69g / Fluid 0 fl oz

Instructions (2 servings)

1. Add all ingredients to a 12 fl. oz , or a larger container with a lid.
2. Stir until it combined.
3. Cover it and set in the fridge for a night (at least 8 hours).
4. The next day, add additional milk until you reach desired consistency.
5. Divide between two little bowls, add toppings, and enjoy.

CONCLUSION

With new diets entering the industry every year, there's no wonder so many feel a sense of overwhelming. Those most popular often become part of a person's lifestyle. Especially once they notice the benefits and results it offers.

Many dieting techniques associate lowering carbohydrates, sugar, and fat intake for weight loss. Of course, reducing intakes of certain foods can achieve weight loss. But, there are many other reasons people choose to diet.

There are many benefits a person can gain from limiting/eliminating certain foods.

Like the vegan keto diet. Or them as separate diets. They both promote weight loss. Yet, they can also help reduce and inhibit medical conditions.

Take the vegan diet as an example of this. Veganism in particular is popular in today's society. This is due to the sustainable benefits it has on the environment as well as the body. The elimination of animal products is sustainable for the planet. But, it also offers many health benefits. From reducing the risk of heart disease to protection against certain cancers. The simple elimination of certain dietary products can have more benefits than you think. Even more so than weight loss.

Combining two diets can be successful for a person to reap extra benefits. Which can be beneficial for the body, medical or environmental concerns.

It is important to take from this book that being vegan is 100% achievable whilst being on the keto diet. Both are restrictive diets. Yet, a person can combine them with the right knowledge and guidance.

There are many plant-based protein substitutes out there for vegan keto dieters to enjoy. Consuming plant-based alternatives will help you sustain the vegan part of the diet. These plant-based foods are a great source of protein and healthy fats. Which is ideal for inhibiting nutrient deficiencies. These nutrients are also perfect for the keto diet requirements.

The vegan keto diet is ideal for those who do not work well with a high-carb diet. And/or those who do not wish to consume animal products. Or, those with existing medical conditions this diet can benefit.

Vegan keto is more of a diet. Whereas intermittent fasting is less of a diet and more of a lifestyle change. Yet, if a person partakes in either of them for long enough, both are more of a lifestyle change.

To sustain the vegan keto diet, it is key to abide by the foods to follow and avoid. For the vegan keto diet in particular, you must consume high-quality plant protein. As well as low carbs and healthy fats in your meals. It may seem that combining the two food restrictive diets will lack a lot of exciting foods. But, that perception is wrong. There is an extensive list of foods that you can choose from.

First it is important to consider protein. A vegan diet often lacks protein if a person does not find protein-packed substitutes. Protein from animals is "complete" protein.

This provides all the essential amino acids a body needs to grow and function well. Plant-based proteins are "incomplete" as they lack enough amino acids. But, over the years there have been many new vegan packed protein options.

Then, you need to take into consideration the recommended carbohydrate intake. This is between 15 and 40 grams per day. It is important to be aware that carbohydrates are not only present in whole grain foods. Many vegetables can be high in carbohydrates too.

Then, for both diets, you should eat as many healthy fats as possible over unhealthy fats. On the vegan keto diet, you should intake around 25% of your calories from plant protein. Then, 70% or more from healthy fats and the rest carbohydrates.

Intermittent fasting methods do not involve any dietary restrictions. It only restricts the times at which a person eats. Thus, sticking to the vegan keto food list is essential. This is key for a person to reap the benefits that the dietary limitations offer.

It's safe to say that not all diets are safe. Nor are they all effective. There are many diets out there that have unsustainable plans, restrictions, and methods. Do not believe everything you see about new diets.

Also do not believe that a safe diet is beneficial for everyone. Even if a diet has lots of evidence to prove its efficacy and safety, some people can still be at risk. This is usually if they have existing health conditions.

The same goes for the diets in this book. We trust in them and their benefits. Yet, we have to state that if you are within the few that may be at risk, you should avoid the diet. If you do wish to partake in any, do seek medical advice first. Whether that be veganism, keto, intermittent fasting, or any combined.

Use this as your guide for starting the vegan keto diet

and/or intermittent fasting. Now you have full knowledge that being 100% vegan on the keto diet is achievable. All whilst intermittent fasting too. So now, you can put this all into practice.

All diets are safe to combine if you wish to use them all together. If you have any more queries or need a companion with you on this lifestyle/diet journey, use this book as your go-to.

Now you have got all the knowledge you need, you can begin and enjoy it.

REFERENCES

Intermittent fasting: Surprising update - Harvard Health Blog (2020)
https://www.health.harvard.edu/blog/intermittent-fasting-surprising-update-2018062914156

Effect of Alternate-Day Fasting Among Metabolically Healthy Obese Adults (2017)
https://jamanetwork.com/journals/jamainternalmedicine/fullarticle/2623528

Dietary restriction normalizes glucose metabolism and BDNF levels, slows disease progression, and increases survival in huntingtin mutant mice (2003)
https://www.ncbi.nlm.nih.gov/pmc/articles/PMC151440/

Intermittent fasting and caloric restriction ameliorate age-related behavioral deficits in the triple-transgenic mouse model of Alzheimer's disease. (2007)
https://europepmc.org/article/med/17306982

Corrigendum to "Alternate day calorie restriction improves clinical findings and reduces markers of oxidative stress and inflammation in overweight adults with moderate asthma" | Request PDF | Free Radical Biology and Medicine (2007)
https://www.researchgate.net/
publication/6513193_Corrigendum_to_Alternate_day_cal
orie_restriction_improves_clinical_findings_and_reduces_
markers_of_oxidative_stress_and_inflammation_in_overwe
ight_adults_with_moderate_asthma

Intermittent fasting vs daily calorie restriction for type 2 diabetes prevention: a review of human findings (2014)
https://www.sciencedirect.com/science/
article/pii/S193152441400200X

Alternate-day fasting in nonobese subjects: effects on body weight, body composition, and energy metabolism (2005)
https://academic.oup.com/ajcn/article/81/
1/69/4607679

Enhanced thermogenic response to epinephrine after 48-h starvation in humans (1990)
https://pubmed.ncbi.nlm.nih.gov/2405717/

Intermittent fasting vs daily calorie restriction for type 2 diabetes prevention: a review of human findings (2014)
https://www.sciencedirect.com/science/
article/pii/S193152441400200X

Glucose tolerance and skeletal muscle gene expression in response to alternate day fasting (2005)
https://pubmed.ncbi.nlm.nih.gov/15833943/

Functional hypothalamic amenorrhea and its influence on women's health (2014)
https://pubmed.ncbi.nlm.nih.gov/25201001/

Sex-Dependent Metabolic, Neuroendocrine, and Cognitive Responses to Dietary Energy Restriction and Excess (2007)
https://academic.oup.com/endo/article/148/9/4318/2502068

International society of sports nutrition position stand: diets and body composition (2017)
https://jissn.biomedcentral.com/articles/10.1186/s12970-017-0174-y

The effectiveness of breakfast recommendations on weight loss: a randomized controlled trial (2014)
https://pubmed.ncbi.nlm.nih.gov/24898236/

Resting energy expenditure in short-term starvation is increased as a result of an increase in serum norepinephrine (2000)
https://pubmed.ncbi.nlm.nih.gov/10837292/

Effects of 8-hour time restricted feeding on body weight and metabolic disease risk factors in obese adults: A pilot study (2018)
https://content.iospress.com/articles/nutrition-and-healthy-aging/nha170036

(PDF) A low-carbohydrate, ketogenic diet to treat type 2 diabetes (2005)
https://www.researchgate.net/publication/

7449608_A_low-carbohydrate_ketogenic_diet_to_treat_type_2_diabetes

The incidence of dementia and intake of animal products: preliminary findings from the Adventist Health Study (1993)
https://pubmed.ncbi.nlm.nih.gov/8327020/

Type of Vegetarian Diet, Body Weight, and Prevalence of Type 2 Diabetes (2009)
https://www.ncbi.nlm.nih.gov/pmc/articles/PMC2671114/

Microalgae: A potential alternative to health supplementation for humans (2019)
https://www.sciencedirect.com/science/article/pii/S2213453018301435

Vitamin B12 in health and disease (2010)
https://pubmed.ncbi.nlm.nih.gov/22254022/

Effects of yeast-derived β-glucans on blood cholesterol and macrophage functionality (2008)
https://www.tandfonline.com/doi/full/10.1080/15476910802604317

Role of yeast cell wall polysaccharides in pig nutrition and health protection (2007)
https://www.sciencedirect.com/science/article/abs/pii/S1871141307001369

Selenium yeast (1986)
https://pubmed.ncbi.nlm.nih.gov/3521441/

The total antioxidant content of more than 3100 foods, beverages, spices, herbs and supplements used worldwide (2010)
https://www.ncbi.nlm.nih.gov/pmc/articles/PMC2841576/

Hemp Seeds Nutrition Facts & Calories
https://nutritiondata.self.com/facts/custom/1352377/1

Nutritional improvement of cereals by sprouting (1989)
https://pubmed.ncbi.nlm.nih.gov/2692609/

Cardiovascular disease mortality and cancer incidence in vegetarians: a meta-analysis and systematic review (2012)
https://pubmed.ncbi.nlm.nih.gov/22677895/

Dietary adherence and acceptability of five different diets, including vegan and vegetarian diets, for weight loss: The New DIETs study (2015)
https://pubmed.ncbi.nlm.nih.gov/26164391/

Using Multicountry Ecological and Observational Studies to Determine Dietary Risk Factors for Alzheimer's Disease (2016)
https://pubmed.ncbi.nlm.nih.gov/27454859/

Beneficial effects of soy protein consumption for renal function (2008)
https://pubmed.ncbi.nlm.nih.gov/18296369/

Whole-Foods, Plant-Based Diet Alleviates the Symptoms of Osteoarthritis (2015) https://www.ncbi.nlm.nih.gov/pmc/articles/PMC4359818/

A multicenter randomized controlled trial of a plant-based nutrition program to reduce body weight and cardiovascular risk in the corporate setting: The GEICO study (2013)
https://hsrc.himmelfarb.gwu.edu/cgi/viewcontent.cgi

Beyond meatless, the health effects of vegan diets: findings from the Adventist cohorts (2014)
https://pubmed.ncbi.nlm.nih.gov/24871675/

Understanding Fiber
https://dtc.ucsf.edu/living-with-diabetes/diet-and-nutrition/understanding-carbohydrates/counting-carbohydrates/learning-to-read-labels/understanding-fiber/

Higher insulin sensitivity in vegans is not associated with higher mitochondrial density (2013)
https://pubmed.ncbi.nlm.nih.gov/24149445/

Soy product and isoflavone intake and breast cancer risk defined by hormone receptor status (2010)
https://pubmed.ncbi.nlm.nih.gov/19860847/

Fruit and vegetable consumption and all-cause, cancer and CVD mortality: analysis of Health Survey for England data (2014)
https://jech.bmj.com/content/68/9/856

Dietary legume consumption reduces risk of colorectal cancer: evidence from a meta-analysis of cohort studies (2015)
https://pubmed.ncbi.nlm.nih.gov/25739376/

(PDF) A Low-Fat Vegan Diet Improves Glycemic Control and Cardiovascular Risk Factors in a Randomized Clinical Trial in Individuals With Type 2 Diabetes | Diabetes Care (2006)
https://www.researchgate.net/publication/6912286_A_Low-Fat_Vegan_Diet_Improves_Glycemic_Control_and_Cardiovascular_Risk_Factors_in_a_Randomized_Clinical_Trial_in_Individuals_With_Type_2_Diabetes

Comparative effectiveness of plant-based diets for weight loss: A randomized controlled trial of five different diets (2014)
https://www.sciencedirect.com/science/article/abs/pii/S0899900714004237

Health effects of vegan diets (2009)
https://pubmed.ncbi.nlm.nih.gov/19279075/

Food Data Central
https://fdc.nal.usda.gov/fdc-app.html

Chia seeds (Salvia hispanica): health promoting properties and therapeutic applications (2017)
https://europepmc.org/article/med/28646829

Mushrooms: a potential natural source of anti-inflammatory compounds for medical applications (2014)
https://pubmed.ncbi.nlm.nih.gov/25505823/

The effect of a low-carbohydrate, ketogenic diet versus a low-glycemic index diet on glycemic control in type 2 diabetes mellitus (2008)
https://www.ncbi.nlm.nih.gov/pmc/articles/PMC2633336/

Beyond Meatless, the Health Effects of Vegan Diets: Findings from the Adventist Cohorts (2014)
https://www.ncbi.nlm.nih.gov/pmc/articles/PMC4073139/

Vegetarian Diets and Weight Reduction: a Meta-Analysis of Randomized Controlled Trials (2016)
https://pubmed.ncbi.nlm.nih.gov/26138004/

Endogenous DNA damage in humans: a review of quantitative data (2004)
https://pubmed.ncbi.nlm.nih.gov/15123782/

(PDF) Short-term fasting induces profound neuronal autophagy (2010)
https://www.researchgate.net/publication/44660575_Short-term_fasting_induces_profound_neuronal_autophagy

Glycogen shortage during fasting triggers liver–brain–adipose neurocircuitry to facilitate fat utilization (2013)
https://www.ncbi.nlm.nih.gov/pmc/articles/PMC3753545/

Intermittent metabolic switching, neuroplasticity and brain health (2018)
https://read.qxmd.com/read/29321682/intermittent-metabolic-switching-neuroplasticity-and-brain-health

Intermittent fasting promotes adipose thermogenesis and metabolic homeostasis via VEGF-mediated alternative activation of macrophage (2017)
https://www.ncbi.nlm.nih.gov/pmc/articles/PMC5674160/

Calorie restriction regime enhances physical performance of trained athletes (2018)
https://www.ncbi.nlm.nih.gov/pmc/articles/PMC5845356/

International Society of Sports Nutrition Position Stand: Diets & Body Composition (2017)
https://ylmsportscience.com/2017/11/08/international-society-of-sports-nutrition-position-stand-diets-body-composition/

Calorie restriction regime enhances physical performance of trained athletes (2019)
https://www.mdpi.com/2072-6643/11/3/489

Refeeding syndrome: what it is, and how to prevent and treat it (2008)
https://www.ncbi.nlm.nih.gov/pmc/articles/PMC2440847/

ACCESS TO THE ONLINE AREA

You will find all sources, updates, links and bonuses on our dedicated page :

fcer.org/vegan-keto-IF-book/

Don't forget to connect to this page with the password « veganketolifestyle » to get access to all the free bonuses.

Did you enjoy the book?
Please take a minute to review it here

Made in the USA
Monee, IL
12 October 2020